Praise for
Beautiful Bones Without Hormones

"This is a practical, how-to book that lists the new bone-building medications available and provides readers with a 14-day healthy, high-calcium diet for vegetarians; and one for the lactose-intolerant, as well. . . . The coup de grace is the cookbook at the book's end. With recipes for the Famous Croque Monsieur Sandwich and Macaroni and Cheese, calcium never looked so good."
—*Publishers Weekly*

"Conquering osteoporosis requires the multi-pronged approach that is thoroughly presented in this book. If enough people followed his advice, Dr. Root's schedule as an orthopedic surgeon would become very thin, indeed."
—from the foreword by Dr. Isadore Rosenfeld, author of
Power to the Patient

"Osteoperosis is a terrible thief, stealing health and independence from women of all ages. Fight back with *Beautiful Bones Without Hormones,* this simple and effective do-it-yourself manual from one of America's most experienced and trustworthy orthopedic surgeons."
—Lisa R. Callahan, M.D., author of *The Fitness Factor* and
medical director of the Women's Sports Medicine
Center, Hospital for Special Surgery

"An eye-opening account of a very serious disease, osteoporosis, by a thoughtful leader in the field."   —Tim McCarver, Fox Sports

"For those of us who have noticed that stairs are taller, that the distance between the bed and the bathroom grows larger every day, that moaning and groaning has become a daily operatic aria, this book is heaven sent. It's very readable and the plans and advice offered are very doable. I doubt if running around a city block is going to become a reality in my life, but two flights of stairs just might. This book has become a fixture on my bedside table."
—Beverly Sills, coloratura soprano and former director
of the New York City Opera

The All-New Natural

Diet and Exercise Program

to Reduce the Risk of

OSTEOPOROSIS

and Keep Your Bones

Healthy and STRONG

GOTHAM
BOOKS

BEAUTIFUL BONES

WITHOUT

HORMONES

Leon Root, M.D.

and BETTY KELLY SARGENT

GOTHAM BOOKS
Published by Penguin Group (USA) Inc.
375 Hudson Street, New York, New York 10014, U.S.A.
Penguin Group (Canada), 10 Alcorn Avenue, Toronto, Ontario, Canada M4V 3B2
(a division of Pearson Penguin Canada Inc.); Penguin Books Ltd, 80 Strand, London WC2R 0RL,
England; Penguin Ireland, 25 St Stephen's Green, Dublin 2, Ireland (a division of Penguin Books Ltd);
Penguin Group (Australia), 250 Camberwell Road, Camberwell, Victoria 3124, Australia (a division
of Pearson Australia Group Pty Ltd); Penguin Books India Pvt Ltd, 11 Community Centre,
Panchsheel Park, New Delhi – 110 017, India; Penguin Group (NZ), Cnr Airborne and Rosedale Roads,
Albany, Auckland, New Zealand (a division of Pearson New Zealand Ltd); Penguin Books
(South Africa) (Pty) Ltd, 24 Sturdee Avenue, Rosebank, Johannesburg 2196, South Africa

Penguin Books Ltd, Registered Offices: 80 Strand, London WC2R 0RL, England

Published by Gotham Books, a division of Penguin Group (USA) Inc.
Previously published as a Gotham Books hardcover edition.

First Gotham trade paperback printing, May 2005

10 9 8 7 6 5 4 3 2 1

Photos © Ian Spanier Photography
Line drawings © Elizabeth Lee Kelly
Two pictures of bone slices © Hospital for Special Surgery, NYC

The Library of Congress has cataloged the Gotham Books hardcover edition as follows:

Root, Leon.
Beautiful bones without hormones : the all-new natural diet and exercise program to reduce the risk
of osteoporosis and keep your bones healthy and strong / Leon Root and Betty Kelly Sargent.
    p.   cm.
  ISBN: 1-592-40062-0 (hardcover : alk. paper)   1-592-40134-1 (pbk.)
  1. Osteoporosis.   2. Osteoporosis—Alternative treatment.   I. Sargent, Betty Kelly.   II. Title.
  RC931.O73 R655 2004
  616.7'16—dc22   2004274306

Printed in the United States of America
Set in Adobe Garamond and Franklin Gothic
Designed by Judith Stagnitto

PUBLISHER'S NOTE

First, foremost, and always, to Paula and our children

LEON ROOT, M.D.

For my children, Elizabeth and James—*beautiful* in every way

BETTY KELLY SARGENT

CONTENTS

FOREWORD   Dr. Isadore Rosenfeld, author of *Power to the Patient*   xi

INTRODUCTION   What Women Should Do to Prevent Osteoporosis Now That the Safety of Hormone Replacement Therapy Has Been Questioned by the Women's Health Initiative Study   xiii

PART ONE
Save Your Bones, Save Your Life   *1*

1. **What *Is* Osteoporosis, Anyway?**   3
2. **Who Is at Risk and Why:** Assessing Your Risk   25
3. **Separating Fact from Fiction:** The Ten Most Important Things You Need to Know to Prevent Osteoporosis   48
4. **The New Bone-Building Medications:** Fosamax, Actonel, Didronel, PTH, and More—Which Ones Work, Which Ones Don't; The Risks, the Benefits; Which Drugs *Not* to Take Together   58

PART TWO
The Dietary Secrets That Can Change Your Life   *71*

5. **The Calcium Revolution:** The Truth About Calcium; Why It Is the Most Important Mineral in Your Body, and the Most Difficult to Absorb   73
6. **Let the Sun Shine In:** How Five to Fifteen Minutes of Sunlight a Day Guarantees All the Essential *Natural* Vitamin D You Need   99

7. **Little Things Mean a Lot:** All About the Other "Must-Have"
    Nutrients to Boost Calcium Absorption   110

8. **The Good, the Not So Good, and the Terrible:** Which Foods
    to Eat; Which to Cut Down On; Which to Avoid Like the Plague   131

9. **The 14-Day, Healthy, High-Calcium Diet; The 7-Day,
    Healthy, High-Calcium Diet for the Lactose-Intolerant;
    The 7-Day, Healthy, High-Calcium Diet for Vegetarians:**
    Healthy Eating Plans to Help You Maximize Calcium
    Absorption—Naturally—from the Foods You Eat   157

10. **The Simple, Long-Term Eating Program to
    Maximize Bone Strength:** Thirty Tips on How to Add
    Calcium to Your Everyday Diet   218

PART THREE
Build Better Bones with Exercise   *225*

11. **Bones Need Exercise Like Babies Need Love:**
    The Simple Weight-Bearing, Muscle-Building Workout
    Program That Guarantees Results   227

12. **The Safest Aerobic and Alternative Therapies:**
    Walking, Swimming, Cycling, Dancing, Yoga, Tai Chi:
    Do They Help?   243

PART FOUR
The Cookbook   *259*

Sixty High-Calcium Recipes   261
The Yummy High-Calcium Cookbook for Kids   308
Resources: Osteoporosis Organizations, Internet Sites,
    Food-Labeling Information, and Support Groups   320
Sources for Help and Information on Related Conditions   323
Glossary   330
Acknowledgments   339
Index   341
Recipe Index   349

FOREWORD

MOST PEOPLE THINK of osteoporosis, the brittle-bone disease, in terms of its end result—fracture. And most orthopedic surgeons, such as Dr. Root, are trained to focus on fixing these breaks. Over the past thirty-five years, during which Dr. Root and I have worked together, he has repaired and other-wise treated more broken bones than anyone else I know. However, it's un-usual and refreshing to find a seasoned orthopedic surgeon, accustomed to dealing with the mechanical complications of osteoporosis, focusing on this disease in the way that counts most—its prevention. For although bone fractures occur suddenly, either spontaneously or as the result of an injury, their real cause is many years in the making. Indeed, as Dr. Root and his co-author, Betty Kelly Sargent, so effectively explain in these pages, the seeds of bony disaster that occur in menopausal women are sown much earlier in life. They bear fruit at an age when the amount of estrogen made by a woman's ovaries begins to taper, causing calcium to seep out of her bones.

However, as Dr. Root emphasizes, there's more to the story than estro-gen and its role in keeping calcium in the bones. The right diet and exercise ensure that calcium enters the bones and stays there.

In this era of fad diets, the consumption of calcium is often inadequate when we're young—and that's the crucial time as far as preventing osteo-porosis is concerned. In an attempt to lose weight, we often avoid dairy products rich in calcium. In this age of couch potato-ism, we spend more time in front of the TV than in the gym or at the park, and we usually don't get enough exercise. Consequently, many women enter menopause with less than optimal amounts of calcium in their bones. Then, when estrogen production dwindles, they become sitting ducks for osteoporosis. Depositing calcium in your bones is like saving money in the bank. The more you accumulate over the years, the more you have when you need it.

This comprehensive book deals with more than general principles. It contains specific information as to what foods are calcium-rich and how much you should consume. Frankly, I never knew Leon was such a maven in the culinary arts. This volume has so many delicious, calcium-rich recipes that it could easily have been titled "Calcium for the Gourmet."

As far as the exercise necessary to prevent osteoporosis is concerned, Dr. Root's expertise is very evident in these pages. That comes as no surprise, since his book *No More Aching Back* has for many years been the bible for millions who suffer from chronic backache.

Finally, Leon shows himself to be the complete physician in that he understands and explains the current controversy concerning the role of HRT in the prevention and treatment of osteoporosis. He is also right on target with the latest medications such as the bisphosphonates, raloxifene, parathyroid agents, and others that are so useful in the prevention, treatment, and even the reversal of this crippling and killing disease.

Conquering osteoporosis requires the multi-pronged approach that is thoroughly presented in this book. If enough people followed his advice, Dr. Root's schedule as an orthopedic surgeon would become very thin, indeed.

—DR. ISADORE ROSENFELD,
AUTHOR OF *Power to the Patient*

INTRODUCTION

OSTEOPOROSIS IS A KILLER. At the very least, it can be a crippler. When your bones become too weak or too brittle to handle the stresses of everyday life, they begin to break down internally and then to just plain break, often when you least expect it. There you are, walking down a sidewalk in February, you slip and fall on a patch of snow-covered ice, and wham, you've fractured your arm and you have to flag down a neighbor to help you back into the house. Or maybe you slip in the shower, twist around to keep from falling, and guess what? You have a broken hip even before you hit the tile. This is often how my patients discover they have osteoporosis. There's no warning, there are no symptoms, they are just going about their lives, doing the things they've done hundreds of times before, and suddenly the smallest fall or misstep occurs and they end up with a broken bone, a fractured hip, a collapsed spine.

Right now, forty-four million people in the U.S. have mild osteopenia, or thinning bones, and 10 million men and women have full-blown osteoporosis. While it is true that women are more susceptible to this condition than men, you might be surprised to learn that one out of every four American men over sixty-five will suffer a broken bone in his lifetime because of osteoporosis, and one third of all men over seventy-five currently have osteoporosis.

We have long known that in women, estrogen helps protect bones. Since osteoporosis is often associated with postmenopausal women, it seems reasonable to assume that the decreasing level of estrogen that accompanies menopause is a primary cause of the problem. Yes and no. Certainly, estrogen plays an important role in keeping our bones healthy, but estrogen is by no means the only route to strong, healthy bones. It is the alternatives to estrogen that I want to concentrate on in *Beautiful Bones without Hormones*.

Here's how it used to work: Often, when women began menopause (somewhere between forty-five and fifty-five) they would also begin a regimen of hormone replacement therapy (HRT). For a long time, HRT was the only U.S. Food and Drug Administration (FDA)–approved drug for the treatment of osteoporosis, and one of its clear benefits is bone health. Other treatments for keeping bones strong included calcium supplements, exercise, and a newer batch of drugs that the FDA later approved for stopping bone loss called bisphosphonates. (I'll discuss these in depth in Chapter 4.) Then, when a recent study by the Women's Health Initiative (WHI) was halted because of evidence that HRT can slightly increase a woman's risk of developing cancer, hundreds of thousands of women stopped taking HRT. It is these women, as well as every American man and woman—especially those over the age of fifty, 55% of whom already have osteopenia—that I want to address and help by writing this book. Incidentally, the FDA now refers to HRT as HT (the word *replacement* has been taken out) and to estrogen replacement therapy (ERT) simply as ET. Because most people are not aware of this change I will continue to refer to them as HRT and ERT.

The good news is that you can prevent osteoporosis, reverse bone loss, strengthen weak bones, and even build new bone naturally—without HRT. The solution lies in understanding how bones are formed and what you need to do to keep them healthy and strong. I'm reminded of the famous line from Julius Caesar, "the fault, dear Brutus, lies not in our stars, but in ourselves." Osteoporosis is almost always fixable if we take the trouble to find out what causes it and what we can do to prevent it. Quite simply, preventing osteoporosis depends on what you eat and what you do. What you need to *eat* is a diet high in absorbable calcium, and I have developed a diet plan that is simple to follow, delicious and provides generous amounts of absorbable calcium every day. What you need to *do* is follow an easy, twenty-minute-a-day, weight-bearing and muscle-building exercise plan to keep both your bones and your body fit and flexible.

My interest in osteoporosis developed as a result of over thirty-five years as a practicing orthopedic surgeon at the Hospital for Special Surgery in New York City, a professor of clinical orthopedics at the Joan and Sanford Weill Medical College of Cornell University, and as the director of the Rehabilitation Department at the Hospital for Special Surgery. I have treated countless patients with collapsing spines, fractured wrists, and broken hips from osteoporosis. I'm sad to say that I've seen many people die from this crippling affliction, deaths that in most cases could have been prevented. I've also seen many treatments for osteoporosis over the years and learned that there is no single magic cure, but if you are willing to take your fate into your own hands by learning about osteoporosis and doing what you need to do to prevent it, you can keep your bones healthy and strong and often even reverse some of the crippling effects of osteoporosis.

In the following chapters I'll tell you everything I've learned about this "silent killer" in my practice. I'll explain just what the disease is and help you evaluate your own risk of developing it. I'll teach you how to separate fact from fiction when it comes to diagnosing and treating the disease, and I'll give you the complete lowdown on all the new and sometimes amazing drugs now on the market, some of which can actually reverse bone loss. I'll let you in on the dietary secrets that I believe can change your life, and I'll give you the simple exercise plan that I follow every day that has kept me standing straight and feeling great for many years.

Keep in mind that if you have or have had any special health problems, you must consult your doctor and seek his or her advice before starting any diet and exercise regimen. Everybody and every body is unique, so it is essential for you to work closely with a doctor who understands your particular medical history and individual needs. I believe that knowledge is power, and I want to share my knowledge with you so that you will have the power to keep your beautiful bones beautiful, to stand tall, to move with grace and ease, and to live a full, rich, and healthy life, a life that otherwise might be compromised by the development of bone-crushing osteoporosis.

—Leon Root, M.D.

PART ONE

SAVE YOUR BONES, SAVE YOUR LIFE

CHAPTER ONE

WHAT *IS* OSTEOPOROSIS, ANYWAY?

W E ARE IN THE MIDST of a global *osteoporosis epidemic,* and most of us don't even know it. For more than one half of the U.S. population over the age of fifty, osteoporosis and low bone mass are a major threat to health and longevity. The fact is that right now, 44 million of us are living with low bone mass (osteopenia, the bone-thinning condition that leads to osteoporosis) or with osteoporosis itself. I was shocked to learn that more than 200 million people worldwide are suffering from this condition, and as the global population continues to age the problem will get even worse. Just take a look at some of these startling statistics recently released by the National Osteoporosis Foundation (NOF):

> **Osteoporosis Fact**
>
> **Osteoporosis-related broken bones affect more women than breast cancer, uterine cancer, and ovarian cancer combined.**

- For the average American woman, the risk of developing osteoporosis is greater than her risk of developing breast cancer and endometrial cancer combined.
- More women die from osteoporosis-related hip fractures each year than from uterine cancer and breast cancer combined. Most of these deaths can be prevented.

○ One out of two women will have an osteoporosis-related bone fracture in her lifetime.

○ One out of every eight men will have an osteoporosis-related bone fracture in his lifetime.

○ **2002:** Forty-four million men and women over fifty in the U.S. are currently suffering from low bone mass, 68% of whom are women.
  • Ten million of these people already have osteoporosis.

○ **2010:** Fifty-two million American men and women over fifty will have low bone mass.
  • Twelve million of these men and women will have osteoporosis.

○ **2020:** Sixty-one million Americans in this age group will have low bone mass.
  • Fourteen million of these people will have osteoporosis.

○ Seventeen billion dollars is spent in the U.S. each year on osteoporosis-related fractures.

○ Osteoporosis is responsible for more than 1.5 million fractures annually, including:
  • 300,000 hip fractures
  • 700,000 vertebral fractures
  • 250,000 wrist fractures
  • 300,000 fractures at other sites

○ Bone health must be considered a top priority for all Americans, as well as everyone over the age of fifty throughout the world.

What I find so disturbing in all this is that so many men and women know so very little about the dangers of osteoporosis. Let me tell you about a patient I have been treating for many years, named Mildred. When she first came to see me she was a feisty, funny, exceptionally bright and alert woman. She was a widow and surrounded herself with friends, most of whom shared her love of working for political causes. Ten years ago, when she was sixty-eight, she fell and broke her wrist. Fortunately, I was able to set the fracture and it healed without complications. Because of her age I suggested she get a bone density test, and much to her surprise, it revealed that she had significant osteoporosis. I urged her to stop smoking, take calcium supplements, and get more exercise. "Thanks," she said. "I appreciate your advice, but I'm just too old for all that." As you might

Osteoporosis Fact

74% of women between the ages of forty-five and seventy-five have never discussed osteoporosis with their doctors.

imagine, things got worse. About two years after the wrist fracture, she fell and fractured her pelvis and lower spine. This time she was hospitalized for four weeks and had to spend three months after that at home, in terrible pain. Finally she was able to walk again, with a cane. This time I was able to get her to stop smoking. Then, about a year and a half later, Mildred slipped on a wet floor, landed on her back and fractured her sacrum and compressed four lumbar vertebrae. Again she was hospitalized for several weeks, and when she was finally allowed to go home, she was confined to bed rest and had to be on constant medication for pain. She was not even able to walk to the bathroom. It was six months before she could leave her home, and she was still in a great deal of pain. By this time she had lost two inches in height, was severely bent over, and could not walk without a walker, much less a cane. Mildred is no longer the lady I knew. She tries to be optimistic, but I can see that this is an enormous effort. She tires easily now, and though she still has a few close friends who help her out, she has had to give up all of her political activities. I mourn the loss of the woman I knew. Osteoporosis was the culprit here, and because she chose to do nothing to treat it, her life will never be the same.

Even more troubling is that most people in the highest risk group, namely postmenopausal women, are not getting adequate information about osteoporosis, nor are they getting advice on how to prevent and treat it. It is estimated that fewer than 30% of women with osteoporosis have been diagnosed with the disease, and of these women, fewer than 15% are receiving treatment. The tragedy is that osteoporosis is usually preventable and treatable, and the earlier you start taking steps to prevent or treat this crippling disease, the better. This is why I strongly recommend that you get a bone density test right now if you are in any of the high-risk groups for osteoporosis. What happened to Mildred need not happen to you. As the saying goes, an ounce of prevention is worth a pound of cure.

There are several types of bone mineral density (BMD) tests available.

Insurance Coverage Tip

As of July 1998, Medicare covers Bone Mineral Density (BMD) tests for:

1. Women over sixty-five, especially those not on estrogen
2. Men and women whose X rays show previous spine fractures
3. Men and women on prednisone or steroids, or who are going to begin such treatment
4. Men and women diagnosed with primary hyperparathyroidism
5. Men and women being treated for osteoporosis to see if therapy is working

---

The tests are simple, painless, and the cost is usually covered by medical insurance. I'll tell you all about who is at risk and why, and describe the types of Bone Mineral Density (BMD) tests in Chapter 2. The sooner you know what your risk factors are, the sooner you and your doctor will be able to decide on the best course of action. In the meantime, the safest and most effective thing that you can do for bone health is to make sure that you're getting lots of calcium in your diet every day. Most people don't get nearly the amount of calcium their bones need each day to stay healthy. I'll tell you how to do it in the following chapters. For now though, if you are over fifty, try to make sure you are getting 1,500 milligrams of calcium in your diet daily. This little step, along with a simple and gentle exercise regimen, will go a long way toward restoring your beautiful bones to optimal health.

Osteoporosis Fact

Osteoporosis is *preventable*.
Osteoporosis is *treatable*.
Osteoporosis cannot be cured.

Prevention is always the best treatment, so talk to your doctor and get a Bone Mineral Density (BMD) test *now* to see what you need to do to keep your bones healthy, strong, and beautiful.

What exactly is osteoporosis? It is "a skeletal disorder characterized by compromised bone strength predisposing to an increased risk of fracture," according to the new definition that the National Institutes of Health came up with in March 2000. It affects our entire skeletal system, and it is characterized by compromised bone strength, which means your bones are less dense than they should be in order to do their three primary jobs: 1) support your body; 2) protect your delicate internal organs, and 3) serve as a storeroom for calcium and other essential minerals you need to stay healthy.

Bone is a living, self-regenerating tissue. It is made up in large part of collagen, a protein giving bone a soft framework, and calcium phosphate, a mineral that makes this framework hard and gives it strength. It is the combination of this protein and mineral that makes bone strong, yet flexible enough to withstand stress. Our body achieves its peak bone mass (maximum bone density and strength) by the time we are between twenty-five and thirty, and it does a pretty good job of keeping bone mass at its peak by working out a precise balance between *resorption,* the removal of old bone, and *formation,* the addition of new bone. When we are children and teenagers, bone is being added faster than it is being removed, but sometime between the age of twenty-five and forty the process starts to reverse, and resorption (removal) slowly begins to exceed bone formation. In other words, our body begins to lose more bone mass than it can replace. Usually, the rate of loss at the beginning of this process is from 0.5 to 1% a year. When resorption occurs too quickly, or formation occurs too slowly, low bone mass starts to occur and, over time, if this imbalance persists, will lead to full-blown, debilitating osteoporosis. Osteoporosis is more likely to develop in people who did not reach optimal bone mass during their bone-building years. Therefore, the prevention of osteoporosis should start as early as in your late teens. Men and women are both affected by this loss, but *when a woman reaches the age of menopause her bone loss accelerates from about 3% up to 7% a year.*

Think of it this way: If you have been diagnosed with low bone mass or density, this means that your bones have less mineral per square inch than they should, when measured against the typical bone mass of a healthy, thirty-year-old Caucasian person. If your diagnosis shows that your bones

Osteoporosis Fact

EVERY HOUR in the U.S.:

- 150 osteoporatic fractures
- 43 deaths from heart attack
- 21 cases of diagnosed breast cancer

Osteoporosis Fact

By the age of seventy to seventy-five, men and women are *equally* at risk of losing bone mass and developing osteoporosis.

Remodeling Cycle of Bone

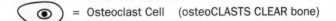 = Osteoclast Cell   (osteoCLASTS CLEAR bone)

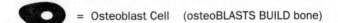 = Osteoblast Cell   (osteoBLASTS BUILD bone)

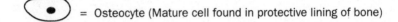 = Osteocyte (Mature cell found in protective lining of bone)

STAGE 1: Resting Phase

• *A protective layer of cells lines the bone*

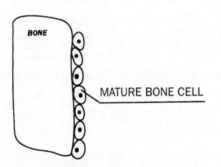

MATURE BONE CELL

STAGE 2: Dissolving Phase

• *Osteoclasts invade*

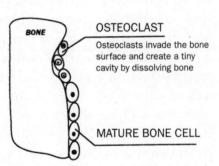

OSTEOCLAST

Osteoclasts invade the bone surface and create a tiny cavity by dissolving bone

MATURE BONE CELL

• *Cavity created*

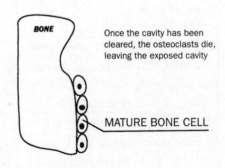

Once the cavity has been cleared, the osteoclasts die, leaving the exposed cavity

MATURE BONE CELL

STAGE 3: Remodeling Phase

• *Osteoblasts assemble*

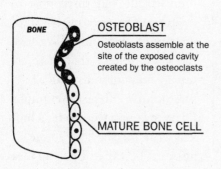

OSTEOBLAST

Osteoblasts assemble at the site of the exposed cavity created by the osteoclasts

MATURE BONE CELL

• *Mineral movement into bone*

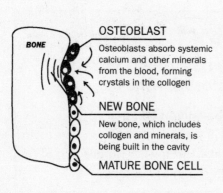

OSTEOBLAST

Osteoblasts absorb systemic calcium and other minerals from the blood, forming crystals in the collogen

NEW BONE

New bone, which includes collogen and minerals, is being built in the cavity

MATURE BONE CELL

STAGE 4: Final Phase

• *Collogen and minerals harden into bone tissue*

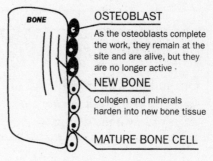

OSTEOBLAST

As the osteoblasts complete the work, they remain at the site and are alive, but they are no longer active ·

NEW BONE

Collogen and minerals harden into new bone tissue

MATURE BONE CELL

• *Osteoblasts become mature bone cells*

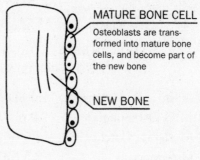

MATURE BONE CELL

Osteoblasts are trans-formed into mature bone cells, and become part of the new bone

NEW BONE

Osteoporosis Facts

T-SCORE

This score compares the bone mineral status of the patient to an average, healthy twenty-five- to thirty-year-old Caucasian subject of the same sex.

Z-SCORE

This score compares the bone mineral status of the patient to that of a person of the same age, sex, and ethnic background.

Osteoporosis Fact

One in four men over the age of sixty-five will break a bone because of low bone density.

are only somewhat less dense than normal, you probably have a condition called osteopenia, meaning that on your bone density test, your T-score was between –1 and –2.5 standard deviations below what your normal bone density was when you were about thirty. On the other hand, if your T-score is below –2.5 you have full-blown osteoporosis. Both of these conditions indicate that the structure of your bone tissue has begun to deteriorate, making your bones more fragile and susceptible to fractures. Osteoporosis is a progressive disease, and as I've said, the scary thing is that there are usually no symptoms until a fracture occurs. Often, for example, I'll be treating a woman for a broken wrist and she'll say to me, "I just can't believe it. I had no idea anything was wrong. Why didn't I have any warning that this could happen? I thought I was perfectly fine." This is why osteoporosis is often referred to as the "silent thief." It just sneaks up on you like a thief in the night and steals from your precious bones.

Osteoporosis Fact

WORLD HEALTH ORGANIZATION STANDARDS FOR DIAGNOSING OSTEOPOROSIS

Normal Bone Mass	1.0 SD (Standard Deviation)
Mild Osteopenia	1.0 to –1.0 (minus 1.0) SD
Moderate Osteopenia	–1.0 (minus 1.0) to –2.5 (minus 2.5) SD
Osteoporosis	–2.5 (minus 2.5) SD or lower

HORMONE REPLACEMENT THERAPY: YES, NO, MAYBE

Before going on about osteoporosis in general, I would like to pause to take a look at the effects of hormone replacement therapy on bone health. Hormone replacement therapy provides women with the female hormones, especially estrogen, that decrease dramatically after menopause. When the hormone estrogen is given alone, it is usually referred to as estrogen replacement therapy (ERT). When estrogen is combined with progesterone (the hormone that prepares the uterus for pregnancy each month) it is generally called hormone replacement therapy (HRT). When a woman reaches *perimenopause,* the transition period leading up to menopause, her hormone levels start to fluctuate, often causing uncomfortable symptoms like hot flashes, mood swings, and interrupted sleeping patterns. Once her hormone levels have fallen dramatically and her periods have stopped for a year, she is considered to be in menopause.

One thing we have known for a while now is that HRT does help prevent bone loss in postmenopausal women. After menopause, when the level of natural estrogen in a woman's body has dropped significantly, her bone loss often accelerates dramatically, to as high as 7% per year, and continues at this rate for the next three to five years. One surefire way to deal with this problem is to replace the estrogen her body was losing with supplemental hormones (HRT). For many years this was the only FDA-approved drug treatment for preventing and treating osteoporosis. Then, in July 2000, when the preliminary results of the federally funded Women's Health Initiative (WHI) study questioned the safety of HRT because of a slight increase in the risk of breast cancer, all bets were off, at least for many of the women taking hormone supplements. In this study, 16,000 randomly selected women, ages fifty to seventy-nine, from all over the U.S., agreed to take part in a long-term effort to learn more about what women can do to stay healthy longer. The study was scheduled to be completed in 2005. The factors to be examined were diet, exercise, calcium supplements, and HRT. The press release in July 2000, which reported a slight increase in the risk of breast cancer, heart attack, and stroke in women on HRT, referred to only the hormone therapy part of the study. The rest of the study is continuing and the results have not yet been announced as of February 2004.

Here's how this particular part of the WHI study worked: Thousands of the participating women were randomly given Prempro, a specific con-jugated estrogen and progesterone combination, which at the time was the most widely used hormone treatment, while the others were given a placebo (a sugar pill). Neither the participants nor the doctors conducting the test knew which women in the study were receiving the hormone and which were receiving the placebo.

The hypothesis for this part of the study was that women taking Prem-pro would show a decrease in coronary heart disease. The researchers also looked at the effect of HRT on breast cancer, stroke, venous thrombosis (blood clotting), colon cancer, and bone fractures.

This study was different from most drug studies because it was designed to help researchers learn about the long-term effects of HRT. Most drug studies look only at the short-term effects of a drug on a particular disease. In other words, the WHI study was designed to try to find out if HRT would help women stay "heart healthy" longer. The minute it became clear that the answer was no, the study would be stopped. The investigators had also agreed that if a significant increase in breast cancer or any of the other sec-ondary diseases they were looking at showed up, the study would be stopped.

After a five-year follow up, the evidence indicated that in 10,000 healthy postmenopausal women who took Prempro for a year, there would be eight more cases of breast cancer (0.08%) than in the similar group not taking Prempro. Looking at the data in this way for the other outcomes, the 10,000 women taking Prempro would have eight extra strokes, eighteen extra pul-monary emboli (blood clots), and seven extra coronary events (heart attacks). However, these same women would have six fewer cases of colon cancer and five fewer bone fractures. There were no differences between the two groups in deaths from any cause. The breakdown would look like this:

According to the WHI Study
Per 10,000 Women on Prempro

THE RISK OF

- Blood clots increased by 18
- Stroke increased by 8
- Breast cancer increased by 8
- Heart attack increased by 7
- Colorectal cancer *decreased* by 6
- Hip fractures *decreased* by 5

DOES THIS MEAN THAT HORMONES ARE BAD?

Not necessarily. Whether or not to take HRT is a highly personal decision based on the medical history and personal philosophy of each and every postmenopausal woman. It is definitely a question that every post-menopausal woman should discuss with her doctor, then weigh the pros and cons and come to her own decision. After the findings of the WHI study, HRT is being prescribed with much more caution these days, but this does not mean that it is absolutely wrong for every woman in every case. What this study showed is that the two products in Prempro should not be given to women to prevent heart disease, stroke, blood clots, or breast cancer. It doesn't mean that they are bad drugs or that they cause these diseases, it simply means that this particular combination of hormones, over time, *may* (according to this study) increase the chances of developing breast cancer, stroke, blood clots, or heart attack. Another study by the National Cancer Institute published in the *Journal of the American Medical Association* in July 2002 showed that women who take estrogen alone, without progestin, were at a high risk of developing ovarian cancer. This study found that taking estrogen (without progestin) for ten years increased the risk of ovarian cancer by 60%. Women who took estrogen alone for twenty years would triple their risk of developing ovarian cancer. On the other hand, some preliminary studies indicated that HRT may be helpful in preventing Alzheimer's disease, though very recently this finding has been disputed. The Nurses' Health Study, an observational study in which tens of thousands of nurses reported on their health and hormone use findings, contradicted some of the findings of the WHI study. The nurses study found that hormone users had a 30% reduction in heart attacks, and that HRT may have a positive effect on macular degeneration, which is an age-related loss of vision. The reason for this discrepancy is still unclear.

What is clear, though, is that there are some positives to hormone therapy. It can relieve the symptoms of menopause, it can keep a woman's skin looking younger, and it helps lower the risk of colon cancer, bone fractures, and perhaps even macular degeneration. But another study of 140,584 women, presented in April 2003 by Dr. Elizabeth Barrett-Connor of the University of California at San Diego, found that when postmenopausal women stopped taking estrogen, they rapidly lost their protection against hip fracture.

Then, on June 25, 2003, a follow-up report on the WHI study was published, and this concluded that compared with women not on hormones, those who take estrogen and progestin tend to develop breast tumors that are harder to spot, and because these tumors are therefore discovered at a more advanced stage, they are harder to cure. In this follow-up study of the 8,506 women on hormones, 199 developed invasive breast cancers, compared with 150 cases in the 8,102 women taking placebos. All of the women in the study had yearly mammograms. Of those using hormones, 25.4% had cancers that had begun to spread to other parts of the body, while this was the case with only 16% of the women taking the placebo. What's more, after one year of treatment, 9.4% of the women in the hormone group had abnormal mammograms, compared with 5.4% in the placebo-taking group.

A second, alarming report found that the combination of estrogen and progestin increased the risk of breast cancer even when the progestin was given in a sequential manner—that is, only on certain days of the month, instead of every day as with Prempro. It had been thought that sequential progestin might be safer than taking it every day, but that no longer appears to be the case. This second report, based on a study directed by Dr. Christopher Li of the Fred Hutchinson Cancer Research Center in Seattle, corroborated the previous finding that women who took estrogen alone had no increased risk of breast cancer, even if they took it for twenty-five years. The problem, though, is that estrogen dramatically increases the risk of uterine cancer, so only women who have had hysterectomies are advised to take unopposed estrogen.

It appears to me that the dangers of HRT have increasingly begun to outweigh the benefits. As I suggested before, what it really comes down to is this: Each woman should talk with a doctor who knows her complete medical history, and together they should decide whether HRT is right for her. Many doctors who formerly advocated the use of HRT now recommend it only for women with very severe symptoms of menopause, such as nearly unbearable hot flashes, and then for only a short period of time. For our purposes here, however, I'm going to talk about how to prevent and treat osteoporosis without hormone therapy, since there is so much controversy about the long-term safety of the hormone medications currently available on the market.

LET'S BONE UP ON BONES

Our skeletons are made up of two types of bone tissue: trabecular bone and cortical bone.

Trabecular bone makes up the interior of the bones of the vertebra, and some is also found in the ends of long bones. It looks like a honeycomb consisting of a system of struts and arches. It is often called "spongy" or "cancellous" bone because of its latticelike structure. Trabecular bone is filled with bone marrow. It accounts for about 20% of the bone in our body, and has a high metabolic rate.

Cortical bone surrounds the trabecular bone and accounts for the remaining 80% of the bone in our bodies. It is solid, dense, and strong, and gives the long bones in our hips, legs, and forearms their strength. It forms the outer layer of the long bones and has a slow metabolic rate so it is broken down and replaced (remodeled) much more slowly than trabecular bone.

If you were to look at a cross section of healthy, dense bone, it would look a little like a latticework, or perhaps Swiss cheese, with lots of solid cheese and a few holes. If you were to look at a cross section of the bone of someone with osteopenia or osteoporosis, it would also look like Swiss cheese, but with lots of holes and very little cheese. From the outside both bones would probably appear to be healthy, but if you were able to see what was going on inside the trabecular part of the second bone, you'd be able to tell right away that the bone is thin, brittle, and weak.

Bone mass and bone density are closely related. When bone mass decreases, bone strength decreases, and fractures are likely to happen with even the slightest amount of external force. Sometimes simply bending over to pick up the newspaper, or even coughing, can cause a fracture.

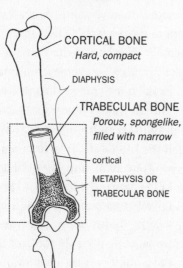

Femur

CORTICAL BONE
Hard, compact

DIAPHYSIS

TRABECULAR BONE
*Porous, spongelike,
filled with marrow*

cortical

METAPHYSIS OR
TRABECULAR BONE

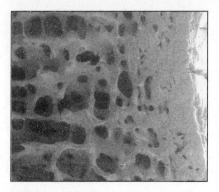 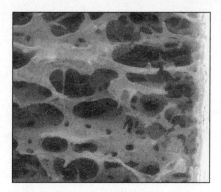

Healthy bone slice   Osteoporatic bone slice

WHY DO BONES BREAK DOWN?

The remodeling process I've been talking about requires the action of two types of bone cells, **osteoblasts** (bone builders) and **osteoclasts** (bone removers). As I've mentioned above, during childhood, the activity of the osteoblasts, the builders, outdoes that of the osteoclasts, the removers, so that young bones can grow in size, weight, density, and strength. Between the ages of twenty-five and thirty our bones have reached their maximum density, and the rapid rate of growth begins to slow down and eventually reverse. Resorption (bone loss) slowly begins to overtake formation, and the gradual process of bone thinning begins. I'll explain more about this in Chapter 5, "The Calcium Revolution," but do remember that one of the best ways to ensure long-term bone health is to make sure that you achieve optimal peak bone mass during the growth years. This means that as a young person you need to have lots of calcium and vitamin D in your diet, and do weight-bearing exercises regularly. Even if you missed out on building healthy bones as a child and teenager, it is never too late to start, but if you are a parent it is important to remember that the stronger the bones your children

Osteoporosis Fact

THE NUMBER OF AMERICANS
AFFECTED EACH YEAR

Osteoporatic Fracture	1,500,000
Heart Attack	500,000
Stroke	225,000
Breast Cancer	184,000
Uterine, Ovarian, and Cervical Cancer	76,000

build today, the longer and healthier their lives are apt to be. We'll talk more about this in the section on Kids and Calcium on page 308.

Osteoporosis Fact

Due to the absence of gravity, astronauts experience bone loss at a rate of about 0.2% per month, even when they engage in two hours of exercise a day.

DIFFERENT TYPES OF OSTEOPOROSIS

Osteoporosis is divided into two basic categories: primary and secondary. Primary osteoporosis occurs when bone loss is due to a problem within the bone itself, usually as the result of a disruption in the normal bone remodeling (removal) cycle. Secondary osteoporosis refers to diseases in other parts of the body that also cause bone loss. In this case the bone loss is secondary to some other disease.

There are three types of primary osteoporosis:

Type I: Postmenopausal osteoporosis (PMO)

Obviously this affects only women, because it is mainly associated with the loss of estrogen that occurs after menopause. It primarily affects the **trabecular** (porous, spongy) bone in the vertebrae and in the wrist, where much of the metabolically active trabecular bone is located. It is because of this type of bone loss that many postmenopausal women will have a spine or wrist fracture within five to ten years of their last menstrual period.

Type II: Age-related osteoporosis (sometimes called senile osteoporosis)

This affects both men and women. It differs from postmenopausal osteoporosis in that bone loss occurs in the

Types of Primary Osteoporosis

Type I: Postmenopausal

Type II: Age-related (or Senile)

Idiopathic:
   Adult
   Juvenile

cortical areas of the skeleton as well as in the trabecular areas. Because of the loss in both types of bone, people with Type II osteoporosis also suffer fractures of the hip as well as the wrist and spine. In women, Type II osteoporosis usually shows up about ten years later than Type I, and it is thought to be caused by calcium and vitamin D deficiency as well as by the age-related changes associated with loss of estrogen and the malfunctioning of the remodeling process.

Idiopathic osteoporosis: adult and juvenile

The word "idiopathic" refers to a disease that arises spontaneously from an unknown or uncertain cause. In other words, doctors do not know the cause of the disease. This is the case with idiopathic osteoporosis.

It is a rare form of primary osteoporosis, and when it occurs in children it is usually around the time of puberty. Fortunately, it often resolves itself after puberty, and the young adult goes on to live a completely bone-healthy life. When idiopathic osteoporosis occurs in adults, the bones become fragile and break, just as they do in people with Type I and Type II osteoporosis. But with these patients, we simply don't know what has caused the disease.

Differences Between Type I and Type II Osteoporosis

	TYPE I	TYPE II
Age	50–75	70 and up
Sex Ratio (F-M)	6:1	2:1
Type of Bone Loss	trabecular	cortical and trabecular
Site of Fracture	spine, wrist	hip, spine, wrist
Rate of Bone Loss	accelerated	slow
Calcium Absorption	decreased	decreased

Secondary osteoporosis is either caused by medications or medical conditions that affect the calcium balance or the microarchitectural integrity of the bones. Fewer than 5% of people with osteoporosis have secondary osteoporosis. Some of its most common causes include:

- **Medications:** corticosteroids, dilantin, phenobarbitol, lithium, aluminum antacids, gonadotropin-releasing hormone agonists, loop diuretics, methotrexate, excessive thyroid medication.

- **Hereditary diseases of the skeleton:** rickets, hypophosphatasia, osteogenesis imperfecta.

- **Endocrine conditions and metabolic diseases:** Cushing syndrome, asicosis, Gaucher's disease, hypogonadism, hyperparathyroidism, Turner's syndrome, Klinefeltner's syndrome, prolactinoma, diabetes mellitus, acromegaly.

- **Other causes:** pregnancy, early surgical menopause (removal of ovaries), exercise-induced amenorrhea, anorexia, bulimia malabsorption, cystic fibrosis, bone marrow diseases including myeloma, mastocytosis, and thalassemia, renal insufficiency, depression, spinal cord injury, systemic lupus hepatic disease, hypercalciuria, and rheumatoid arthritis.

Treating secondary osteoporosis is more complicated than treating primary osteoporosis because you also have to consider the treatment for the underlying disease. If you have secondary osteoporosis, be sure to find a doctor who knows a lot about your primary disease as well as osteoporosis.

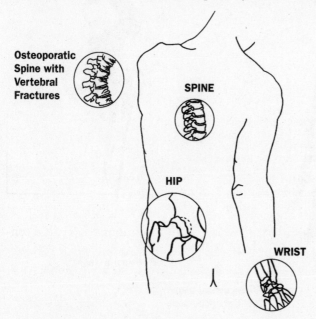

Osteoporatic
Spine with
Vertebral
Fractures

SPINE

HIP

WRIST

Why We Get Osteoporosis

Osteoporosis, which literally means "porous bones," is a degenerative disease. It is not necessarily a "normal part of aging," and it is not limited to postmenopausal women. What happens is that when our body stops getting the calcium that it needs (which does tend to happen more as we get older) it steals the needed calcium from our bones. Over a period of time, when our bones have lost more calcium than they can replace, osteopenia (thinning of the bones) develops. If not treated, this turns into full-blown osteoporosis. One way to look at this is that the process that leads to osteoporosis (calcium being leeched from bones) is actually the long-term negative result of a short-term coping mechanism. The secret to preventing osteoporosis is to give your body all the calcium (and vitamin D and exercise) it needs, so that it doesn't have to start this calcium-stealing process in the first place.

Your body cannot survive without adequate levels of calcium, magnesium, phosphorous, and sodium. When the levels of these minerals and nutrients get too low in your blood, your bones (where these substances are normally

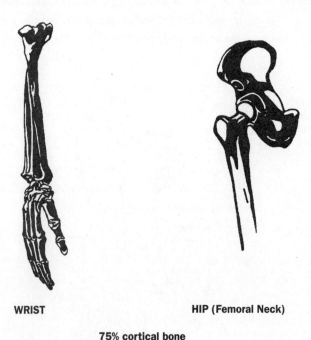

WRIST   HIP (Femoral Neck)

75% cortical bone
25% trabecular bone

stored) give them up to restore a healthy balance of them in your bloodstream. When your blood mineral levels are restored to normal, your body can go on functioning in a healthy way. Think of your bones as your favorite charity. Bones are givers. The most charitable of all our bones are those that have a high trabecular content, like the jaw, pelvis, wrist, and spine. Sometimes the first sign of systemic bone loss is receding gums. The wrist and vertebrae also tend to fracture before the hip, because they are composed largely of trabecular bone, while the hip has a thin outer layer of cortical bone.

Contributing factors that make the development of osteoporosis more likely include lifelong patterns of inadequate nutrition, smoking, alcohol abuse, minimal exercise, depression, some medications, irregular periods, some surgeries, and exposure to toxins in the environment.

Let's take a look at some of the recent statistics on osteoporosis in the U.S. and worldwide.

IN THE UNITED STATES

In the United States, the highest percentages of osteoporosis occur in California, Florida, New York, Pennsylvania, and Texas. It is not surprising that these states also rank high in the proportion of older residents.

Here are some more interesting statistics about the lifetime fracture risks for Americans:

○ After the age of fifty, Caucasian women have a 40% chance of fracturing their wrist, hip, or spine in their lifetime, specifically:

18% chance of hip fracture

16% chance of spine (vertebral) fracture

16% chance of wrist fracture

This is equal to the *combined* risk of developing breast, uterine, and ovarian cancer in the remaining years of their lives

(Source: Melton, Chrischilles, Cooper, Lane, and Riggs, 1992)

○ After the age of fifty, Caucasian men have a 13% risk of osteporatic bone fracture, specifically:

6% chance of hip fracture

4% chance of spine fracture

3% chance of wrist fracture

(Source: Melton et al., 1992)

○ For African-Americans, data is currently only available for the hip. The lifetime risk factor is:
  5.6% for women
  2.8% for men

(Source: Cummings, Black and Rubin, 1989)

These statistics are still being refined and will be discussed in more detail in the next chapter.

States with the Highest Percentages of Osteoporosis	
California	14
Florida	14
New York	14
Pennsylvania	14
Texas	13

(Source: National Osteoporosis Foundation, 1997)

WHAT ARE THE COSTS ASSOCIATED WITH THESE OSTEOPORATIC FRACTURES IN THE U.S.?

○ $38 million per day

○ $13.8 billion per year
  • 62% inpatient care
  • 28% nursing home care
  • 10% outpatient care

Hip fractures account for about 63% of these costs and fractures at other sites for the remaining 37%.

(Source: Ray, Chan, and Thamer, 1997)

WORLDWIDE STATISTICS

It is interesting to see some of the worldwide statistics for the incidence of hip fractures related to osteoporosis:

Yearly Hip Fracture Rates Per 100,000 People Thirty-five and Older	WOMEN	MEN
USA (Rochester, MN)	319.7	177.0
USA (District of Columbia)		
Whites	231.8	82.0
Blacks	118.8	109.7
Finland	212.8	136.1
Norway (Oslo)	421.1	230.5
Sweden (Malmo)	237.2	101.4
Holland	187.2	107.9
United Kingdom (Oxford, Dundee)	142.2	69.2
Israel (Jerusalem)		
American/European-born	201.8	113.9
Native-born	168.0	107.5
Asian/African-born	141.7	109.2
Hong Kong	87.1	73.0
Singapore (total)	42.1	73.1
Indian	312.9	131.4
Chinese	59.0	106.1
Malay	24.2	35.4
New Zealand		
Whites	220.4	98.6
Maori	104.4	84.0
South Africa (Johannesburg)		
Whites	256.5	98.8
Bantu	14.0	14.3

(Source: Adapted from Melton et al., 1983)

As the world population ages, the risk of a worldwide osteoporosis epidemic grows. People are living longer now, and the fastest-growing segment of the population is the oldest of the old, those people eighty-five and up. By the year 2050, the incidence of hip fracture will increase fourfold, from 1.66 million fractures in 1990 to 6.26 million fractures in 2050. The most significant increase is expected in Asia. Today, Asia accounts for 30% of all hip fractures. By 2050, Asia is expected to account for 50% of all hip fractures.

WHAT DOES THIS HAVE TO DO WITH ME?

There is simply no question that we are facing a worldwide osteoporosis epidemic in the near future, and it is likely to affect you or someone you care about. Part of the reason that this is such a tragedy is that osteoporosis is frequently preventable and always treatable. My goal is to help you better understand this crippling disease. Right now, you can start taking the three simple steps to prevent this killer disease:

1. **Eat right**—to get adequate calcium and vitamin D into your diet.
2. **Exercise**—to keep your bone density at its maximum.
3. **Get a BMD test** if you are in any of the high-risk groups for developing osteoporosis.

Prevention requires some concentrated effort on your part, but the payoff is enormous. Think of it. You can probably add years of healthy, active, pain-free living to your already increased life expectancy by making a few simple changes in your lifestyle. Even if you already have osteoporosis, there is so much you can do to treat it, and the prognosis is better now than it ever has been before. You can do it. You can live a healthier, happier, longer life. It is never too late to learn. It is never too late to begin.

CHAPTER TWO

———— ▬▬▬ ————

WHO IS AT RISK
AND WHY

Assessing Your Risk

T HE SIMPLE FACT is that we are all at risk of developing osteoporosis, but for some of us the risk is greater than for others. A major survey, sponsored by the International Osteoporosis Foundation (IOF) in June 2000, found that despite the new research and education on osteoporosis available worldwide, it is still not being detected early enough to protect postmenopausal women from osteoporosis-related bone fractures. "Although nearly 100% of doctors and women recognize that osteoporosis is a serious health threat," said Dr. Pierre Delmas, the president of the IOF, "women appear to be leaving the doctor's office with a limited understanding of their personal risk, and as a result, are doing very little to protect their bones. Much work remains to be done by women and doctors alike." He went on to point out that women's understanding of their personal risk is alarmingly low. Even though one in two postmenopausal women will be affected by osteoporosis, a shocking 85% do not believe that they are personally at risk of developing the disease. What's more, while 65% of doctors reported that they routinely do health-status reviews among their postmenopausal patients, only 20% of the patients recalled having been screened for osteoporosis. Among the women already suffering from osteoporosis, 80% said they had no awareness of the risk factors before they developed the disease, and one third of these women reported that they were not currently taking medication to help prevent fractures. The study concluded that it is urgent for doctors to commit to making their patients over fifty aware of the risk factors of the disease and to test them when necessary.

And it is equally imperative that all postmenopausal women take the initiative in discussing osteoporosis with their doctors, and ask direct questions about what preventive measures they might take.

The good news is that breakthroughs in the diagnosis and treatment of osteoporosis are being made all the time. On November 3, 2003, Sharon Begley, reporting for *The Wall Street Journal,* announced the discovery of a gene, some versions of which "triple a person's risk of developing osteoporosis, and bone-related fractures." The discovery was made by Kari Steffansson, the founder of deCode Genetics in Reykjavic, Iceland, and published in a new journal called *PloS Biology.* What the study found is that a gene called BMP2, which stands for bone morphogenetic protein 2, apparently affects the activity of the osteoblasts (the bone builders) and so has an impact on bone formation. Dr. Steffansson believes that this gene affects the peak bone mass we achieve when we are young adults.

There are apparently three forms of this BMP2 gene that put a person in the high-risk category for developing osteoporosis. DeCode Genetics is currently working on a DNA-based kit for diagnosing those at risk. But being at high risk genetically does not necessarily mean that you will develop osteoporosis. All it means is that you should be especially vigilant in making sure that you get adequate calcium and vitamin D in your diet, that you should exercise religiously, and that you should carefully monitor your bone density with BMD testing, so that if a problem does crop up, you can begin treating it right away, before it becomes serious.

Before I begin discussing the risk factors that you can and cannot change, I suggest you take this little quiz to see where you stand in the risk department. Circle yes or no on the following questions:

Assessing Your Risk

1. I am female	Yes	No
2. I am over fifty	Yes	No
3. I am Caucasian, Asian, or Hispanic	Yes	No
4. I have a small frame, or I am thin for my body type	Yes	No
5. I have a family history of osteoporosis	Yes	No
6. I am postmenopausal	Yes	No

7. I had menopause early (before forty-five) or had my ovaries removed before fifty	Yes	No
8. I have been taking high doses of thyroid medication or cortisone-based drugs (steroids)	Yes	No
9. I am a smoker	Yes	No
10. I consume more than three glasses of alcohol, two cups of coffee (caffeinated), or soft drinks (caffeinated) a day	Yes	No
11. I am fairly inactive, physically	Yes	No
12. I have anorexia nervosa	Yes	No
13. My diet is low in calcium	Yes	No
14. I have amenorrhea (absence of normal menstrual periods)	Yes	No
15. I have had a broken bone after forty	Yes	No
16. I have lost more than one inch in height	Yes	No
17. I have frequent diarrhea (caused by celiac, Crohn's, or other disease)	Yes	No
18. I am male and suffer from impotence or other symptoms related to low testosterone	Yes	No

Now add up the yes answers to get your risk score. If you have answered yes to seven or more of the questions, your risk of developing osteoporosis or osteopenia is high. If you have answered yes to between four and seven questions, your risk is moderate. And if your yes answers are between zero and three your *current* risk is low.

Let me remind you again that even if your risk of developing osteoporosis is high or moderate, that doesn't mean that you will necessarily develop the condition. What it does mean is that you should get a BMD test right away, because if you are at risk now the risk will only increase as you

My Osteoporisis/ Osteopenia Risk

High (7–15)
Moderate (4–7)
Low (0–3)

get older. As I will say over and over, osteoporosis is usually preventable and always treatable, but it is not curable. Why even flirt with the possibility of developing this crippling condition when there is so much you can do to prevent it?

RISK FACTORS YOU *CANNOT* CHANGE

O Age

O Gender

O Body size

O Ethnicity

O Family history

O Diseases causing secondary osteoporosis

AGE

The older we get, the higher our risk of developing osteopenia or osteoporosis. Here's how it works. We all tend to lose a little bone mass density (usually between 0.5% and 1.0% per year) after the age of thirty. Then, because of the sudden loss of estrogen after menopause, the risk of developing osteoporosis becomes much greater for women than for men—for a while, that is. This discrepancy lasts for about five years after menopause, but by the time both men and women have reached seventy-five, the risk is equal for both sexes. Approximately 30% of American women over fifty have osteoporosis, and more than 50% of women over eighty have it. In fact, a woman's risk of developing osteoporosis doubles every five years after menopause, and one in six women will have an osteoporotic hip fracture in her lifetime.

There are two reasons that age has a negative effect on our bone health. First, as I've explained, as we age things begin to slow down. Bone loss begins to outpace bone formation, taking away more bone than our body is able to replace, and we are left with weakened, thinning, fragile, brittle bones. Second, as our metabolism begins to slow down and work less efficiently, it becomes more difficult for us to absorb the natural bone-building calcium in our diet, so our already weakened bones become starved for calcium and become even weaker. When we were adolescents, our intestines were able to absorb about 75% of the calcium we ingested. As adults, the absorption level usually falls to about 50%, and by the time we are elderly we are absorbing only about 30% of the calcium in our diet. So the combination of impaired calcium absorption and increased bone loss does not bode well for strong, healthy bones. One early study from the Mayo Clinic looked at men and women from age twenty to eighty-nine. The study found that during a woman's lifetime, she could expect to lose about 47% of the bone

> ## Exercise and Age
>
> Women who start exercising after 65 reduce their risk of premature death by 48%, according to a new study that followed 7,500 women over a twelve-year period.

density in her spine and 39% in her wrist. Men of equivalent age would lose only 14% from their spine and an insignificant amount from the wrist. By the age of sixty-five, half the women in the study had lost enough bone to be at risk for a fracture, and by eighty-five they were all at risk. Several later studies have suggested that bone loss for women may begin in their thirties, even earlier than we had thought. Further research also indicates that bone loss from the hips may begin for both men and women in their late thirties.

Most medical professionals believe that just as the loss of estrogen has a negative effect on bone health in women, loss of testosterone in men works much the same way. The difference is that soon after menopause, both estrogen and testosterone loss are dramatic in women, whereas in men this process is usually more gradual. For Type I primary osteoporosis, the high-risk age for women is roughly between fifty and seventy-five. For Type II primary osteoporosis, the high-risk age for both men and women is seventy and beyond. Primary idiopathic osteoporosis can strike anyone at any age, but fortunately it is very rare and often cures itself, especially in pubescent children.

Another reason that age is a risk factor in osteoporosis is that as we get older, all of the other risk factors have more time to do their work. The longer we are calcium deficient, the more damage is done to our bones. The same is true with estrogen deficiency. Furthermore, we generally become less physically active as we get older, and this, too, has a negative effect on our bones.

Still another aspect of our waning ability to absorb calcium is that our skin and kidneys do not make vitamin D as efficiently as they once did. This vitamin D deficiency further cuts down on our ability to absorb the calcium we put into our digestive systems. Then, too, after the age of about sixty most of us experience a decline in the stomach acid we need to absorb calcium, so it is easy to see why we can develop a significant calcium deficiency even though we may never have had an absorption problem before. All this, combined with the fact that our production of osteoblasts (bone builders) is slowing down—so that the bone that is being removed by the osteoclasts (bone clearers) is not being adequately replaced—can lead to a serious and seemingly sudden overall loss of bone, unless we start taking the time to educate ourselves on just how to reverse these conditions.

As far as I know, there is not much we can do to stop getting older (although as many of my friends have pointed out, getting older sure beats the alternative), but there is a lot we can do to stay healthy as we age. In fact, getting older is good. Just don't get *old!* We can make sure that we get adequate calcium into our bodies, and we can take the steps necessary to make sure that our bodies can absorb the calcium they need. By eating right, taking calcium supplements when necessary, exercising, and getting enough vitamin D, we can help ourselves enormously. I have been a major advocate of proper diet, exercise, and a healthy lifestyle since I began my medical practice, and the older I get the more convinced I am that most of us can remain healthy, active, and productive into our eighties and even nineties if we are willing to start taking the simple steps necessary right now. So, although age is clearly one of the risk factors that you can't change, it most certainly is one you can work with.

GENDER

There is no question that your chances of developing osteoporosis are greater if you are a woman, especially before the age of seventy. As I've already explained, Type I primary osteoporosis is specific to postmenopausal women, due to their loss of estrogen. The National Osteoporosis Foundation (NOF) estimates that almost 80% of Americans with osteoporosis are women.

There are actually three reasons why women are more susceptible to osteoporosis than men. One is estrogen loss at menopause. In the first five years after menopause, women experience a rapid increase in bone loss, going from 1% per year to as high as 7% per year. This is why it is not unusual for a postmenopausal woman to lose 15 to 25% of her bone mass over a five-

Hip Fracture Fact

24% of hip fracture patients over fifty die within the year following the fracture.

NOF Figures for Americans over Fifty			
	2002	**2010**	**2020**
Women with low bone mass or osteoporosis	29,600,000	35,100,000	40,900,000
Men with low bone mass or osteoporosis	14,100,000	17,300,000	20,500,000

year period. Some women lose up to 35% of their bone mass in those five years. For most women, this rapid loss begins to slow down by the age of sixty to sixty-five, but serious damage has often already been done.

The second factor that makes women more vulnerable to bone loss is that they tend to build less bone when they are young than men do. Boys are frequently more athletic than girls, and they often engage in more vigorous exercise, so boys and young men tend to build more bone in their early life. Boys and men are also gener-

Hip Fracture Fact

The rate of hip fracture is two to three times higher in women than men. However, the one-year mortality rate following the fracture is almost twice as high in men as in women.

ally taller and heavier than girls and women, and this gives them yet another advantage in the bone-health department. Third, girls often become calcium-deficient as teenagers, while boys frequently have an adequate intake of calcium well into their twenties.

By the time men and women reach the age of seventy, the rate at which their bodies lose bone is about equal, so the risk of developing osteoporosis is about the same.

BODY TYPE

If you are female, petite, fair-skinned, or small-boned for your size, or if you are tall but relatively thin (weighing 127 pounds or less, according to most researchers), you run a fairly high risk of developing osteoporosis. There is not much you can do about your body size except to educate yourself on the

Body-Type Risk Factor

Tall, thin, fair-skinned women have a high risk of developing osteoporosis.

Weight Risk Factor

Sudden weight loss after menopause, (more than 10% of your body weight) can *double* your chances of developing osteoporosis. If you need to lose weight after menopause, do it slowly and under the care of your doctor.

risks associated with your particular frame and to make sure you get a lot of absorbable dietary calcium and exercise. When it comes to osteoporosis, this is one time that weight works in your favor. We live in a skinny-obsessed society, in which it is estimated that at any given time, at least 40% of us are on some kind of diet. My advice is that if you are a woman and you are overweight, try to lose that weight before menopause. If you wait until after menopause and lose a lot of weight quickly, you greatly increase your risk of developing osteoporosis. However, if you do decide to lose weight during or after menopause, try to do it slowly and, if possible, under a doctor's care. It can be safe if you do it right, making sure that you get lots of exercise and generous amounts of absorbable calcium into your diet.

ETHNICITY

Significant risk has been reported in people of all ethnic backgrounds, but Caucasian and Asian women and men run the highest risk of developing osteoporosis. Hispanic and African-American women and men have a lower, but still serious risk. Here is an approximate breakdown for men and women, according to figures from the National Osteoporosis Foundation:

Women

- 80% of all Americans affected by osteoporosis are women

- 5% of African-American women over fifty have osteoporosis
  - 35% of them have low bone mass

○ 10% of Hispanic women over fifty have osteoporosis
 • 49% of them have low bone mass

○ 20% of non-Hispanic white and Asian women over fifty have osteoporosis
 • 52% of them have low bone mass

Men

○ 20% of all Americans affected by osteoporosis are men

○ 7% of non-Hispanic white and Asian men over fifty have osteoporosis
 • 19% of them have low bone mass

○ 3% of Hispanic men over fifty have osteoporosis
 • 23% of them have low bone mass

These figures are estimates, and we don't know for sure why the differences occur in the various groups.

Right now, 300,000 African-American women have osteoporosis. Somewhere between 80% and 95% of bone fractures suffered by the women in this group who are over sixty-four years old are osteoporosis related. More African-American women are likely to die after a hip fracture than women in the other groups. As African-American women get older, their risk of hip fracture doubles about every seven years. Diseases prevalent in the African-American population, such as sickle-cell anemia and systemic lupus, are also linked to osteoporosis, making secondary osteoporosis more likely. Recent studies show that the average African-American woman consumes 50% less calcium than the Recommended Dietary Allowance. An additional problem is that as many as 75% of adult African-Americans are lactose

European Union

• 40% of middle-aged women and 15% of middle-aged men will suffer an osteoporatic fracture in their remaining lifetime.
• Every thirty seconds someone in the EU has an osteoporosis-related fracture.
• Osteoporosis will double in the next fifty years.
• Only half of all osteoporotic fractures are diagnosed.

Bone Fracture Fact

Caucasian women sixty-five and older have twice the incidence of fractures as African-American women.

intolerant, so it is difficult for them to get the calcium they need from calcium-rich milk, yogurt, and dairy products. We will discuss lactose intolerance in Chapter 9, but the good news is that a recent study found that many people with lactose intolerance can actually digest as much as two cups (16 oz.) of milk a day if they divide it into small servings spread out throughout the day.

Hispanic women also run a significant risk of developing osteoporosis. According to the National Health and Nutrition Examination Survey (NHANES III), between 300,000 and 400,000 Mexican-American women over fifty have a significant loss of bone density. About 100,000 of them

Osteoporosis Facts Worldwide

- Worldwide, osteoporosis affects more than 200 million people.
- Worldwide, osteoporosis affects one in three women over fifty and one in eight men.
- In the Middle East, the number of hip fractures will triple in the next twenty years.
- Asia will have the most dramatic increase in hip fractures over the next twenty years due to a growing population and changing lifestyle.
- Worldwide, hip fractures are estimated to rise from 1.7 million in 1990 to 6.3 million by 2050.
- Every thirty seconds in Europe, someone suffers an osteoporosis-related hip fracture.
- In Europe there are more than 480,000 hip fractures every year, up 25% in the last three years.
- Osteoporosis fractures are likely to double in the next half-century.
- Probably less than half the women who have osteoporosis have been diagnosed in France, Germany, Italy, the United States, and the United Kingdom.

(13–16%) already have osteoporosis. Like Caucasian and African-American women, they consume less calcium than the Recommended Dietary Allowance, in all age groups. What's more, it is estimated that the number of hip fractures worldwide will increase sharply over the next fifty years, especially in Asia and Latin America. The Hispanic population in the United States is growing faster than the non-Hispanic population. Between 1980 and 1990 it increased by 53%, compared with only 6.7% for non-Hispanics. The Bureau of Census estimates that the Hispanic population will almost triple between 1995 and 2050, and as this population ages, the number of Hispanic people with osteoporosis will soar. Worldwide, the number of elderly is increasing most rapidly in Africa, Asia, Latin America, and the Middle East. These areas will account for 70% of the 6.26 million hip fractures expected in the year 2050. In fact, the worldwide incidence of hip and other osteoporosis-related fractures will increase fourfold over the next fifty years, and the cost of care will threaten the viability of the healthcare systems in many of these countries, according to B. L. Riggs and L. J. Melton in their report, "The Worldwide Problem of Osteoporosis." As they put it, "Unless decisive steps for intervention are taken now, a catastrophic global epidemic of osteoporosis seems inevitable."

FAMILY HISTORY

If you have a family history of osteoporosis, then, as with so many conditions, your risk of getting it goes up. Let's say your mother had a broken hip. This suggests that your risk factor (remember we are only talking about risk here, not actuality) would double. It is estimated that if someone in your immediate family has primary osteoporosis, you have between a 60% and 80% chance of developing the disease yourself. Why is it important to assess your family history? Because when you understand that your risk factor is high, you know how important it is to get a BMD test and stay on top of your bone health long before you have any signs of trouble.

RISK FACTORS YOU *CAN* CHANGE

- BMD testing
- Lack of exercise

O Smoking

O Alcohol

O Caffeine

O Low calcium and vitamin D

O Low body weight

O Certain medications

Obviously, there are some risk factors you simply can't do much about, but there are a host of others that you can. I'm not suggesting that it is easy to change the patterns of a lifetime, or that you can simply stop taking necessary medications because they enhance your risk of developing osteoporosis. I just feel that it is important to be aware of these factors so that you can deal with them in your own way, in your own time, and as effectively as possible. Here is a list of some of the risk factors you *can* change.

BMD TESTING

I simply cannot overemphasize how important it is to get a BMD test if you have even one or two risk factors for osteoporosis. As I've mentioned before, most of the tests are now covered by medical insurance, and there is no substitute for taking early prevention measures if you are even at the slightest risk of developing osteoporosis. Talk to your doctor. See what he or she recommends. With my patients I generally recommend testing for:

O All women, forty or older who have had a bone fracture

O All postmenopausal women under sixty-five who have one or more additional risk factors besides menopause, including a history of fracture as an adult, being Caucasian, having impaired eyesight despite correction, having a history of alcoholism, smoking, or low dietary intake of calcium, or taking certain medications

O All women sixty-five or older regardless of risk factors

O All men seventy or older

○ All men, women, and children who have known secondary causes of osteoporosis

There are several types of BMD tests, and I have described them on pages 44–46. All the tests are simple, painless, and usually paid for, at least in part, by your medical insurance.

LACK OF EXERCISE

As you well know by now, I am a big believer in exercise, not only as a safeguard against osteoporosis but as a good way to help stay happier and healthier, longer. Without weight-bearing activity, bones become thin and weak. We see this often in patients who are confined to prolonged bed rest. Sometimes it takes months for them to recover their strength. Even plaster casts that are put on to stabilize broken bones and help them heal can, ironically, promote bone loss. One study found that when a patient wore a wrist cast for as little as three weeks, 6% of the bone in that area was lost. I'll go into the specific exercise regimen I recommend in Chapter 11, but for now just remember that even modest weight-bearing exercise can go a long way toward saving your beautiful bones.

SMOKING

Smoking is a real no-no when it comes to osteoporosis. We all know about the many terrible things that smoking can do to you, but be assured that smoking is really bad for your bones. I've explained that estrogen helps prevent osteoporosis by inhibiting the action of osteoclasts, the cells that clear away bone. Smoking has the effect of inactivating estrogen, leaving the smoker with what amounts to an estrogen deficiency. Women who smoke usually reach menopause before women who don't. Not only that, smokers are often less physically active than nonsmokers, which again increases the risk of developing osteoporosis. Nobody said it would be easy, but if you can possibly stop, or even cut back on smoking, you'll be doing a great service to your bones, as well as your lungs and your health in general.

ALCOHOL

Americans consume the equivalent of 500 million gallons of pure alcohol each year, according to *Prevention's Giant Book of Health Facts.* Moderate drinking is fine, but excessive use of alcohol can be very dangerous for your bones. More than three drinks a day can have a negative impact on bone health. Here's what we know about the effects of alcohol on healthy bones:

1. **Alcohol disrupts our calcium balance.** Parathyroid hormone (PTH) and vitamin D regulate the balance of calcium in our systems. Exposure to alcohol elevates our PTH levels and puts a strain on our calcium reserves. Chronic alcohol abuse, which causes continuous elevation in PTH, can cause a secondary condition known as hyperparathyroidism, the effects of which further deplete the calcium we have stored in our bones. Alcohol also inhibits the production of enzymes found in the kidney and liver that convert the inactive form of vitamin D into its active form, thus interfering with the absorption of calcium. Vitamin D deficiency can also lead to *osteomalacia,* a bone condition associated with fractures, pain, and even deformity. Excessive alcohol also increases magnesium excretion in the urine, which in turns makes calcium absorption difficult.

2. **Alcohol has a negative effect on our hormones.** In men excessive alcohol reduces testosterone, thereby decreasing the activity of osteoblasts, the cells that make new bone. In premenopausal women, chronic alcohol exposure can lead to irregular menstrual periods, thereby further increasing the risk of osteoporosis.

3. **Moderate alcohol use may have a positive affect on bone health in postmenopausal women.** This may come as a big surprise to you. The reason for this is that alcohol increases the conversion of testosterone into *estradiol,* a hormone often used to prevent bone loss after menopause. I'm certainly not suggesting that postmenopausal women take up drinking in a big way, but it is interesting to note that a glass or two of wine a day may actually be beneficial to bone health. There is no evidence, however, that moderate drinking is beneficial to bone density in premenopausal women or in men. Sorry about that!

4. **Excessive alcohol increases the level of cortisol.** This is a corticosteroid that, at high levels, leads to decreased bone formation and in-

creased bone resorption (breakdown). Corticosteroids diminish calcium absorption, and this leads to increased PTH secretion, which then causes further bone loss.

5. **Alcohol appears to have a toxic effect on osteoblasts (bone builders), suppressing bone formation.** Osteoclasts (bone clearers), which are responsible for bone breakdown or remodeling, may be stimulated by exposure to alcohol. Most heavy drinkers have significant bone loss.

6. **Excessive alcohol increases the risk of bone fracture.** The reason for this is obvious. Intoxicated people often have impaired balance and fall frequently, breaking wrists, hips, even vertebrae. The older we get, the greater the risk of fractures resulting from excessive drinking.

7. **The abstinence cure.** There is some good news in all of this. Studies show that when an alcohol-addicted person stops drinking completely, he or she experiences a rapid recovery of osteoblast function. It even appears that bone loss may be partially restored when the alcohol abuse is stopped.

8. **Poor nutrition.** Frequently, people who drink excessively don't bother with a well-balanced diet, and this of course leads not only to a calcium deficiency but to many other health problems as well. If you are a heavy drinker, it is most important to get a BMD test now.

CAFFEINE

Since caffeine is a diuretic to the kidneys, it increases the amount of calcium excreted in urine. Even though caffeine occurs naturally in the seeds, leaves, or fruits of sixty-three different plants, it has chemical, druglike effects on the body. It is a stimulant to the brain and heart, as so many of us know from experience when we find that we can't really get going until after we've had our first cup of coffee in the morning. Caffeine is most often found in tea leaves, cola nuts, cola beans, and coffee beans, and as with alcohol, it is fine when used in moderation, but can have a negative effect on our bones when we overdo it.

Every day, we lose between 100 and 250 mg of calcium through the kidneys into the urine. My feeling is that anything that increases calcium loss in the urine, which caffeine does, simply leads to increased calcium deficiency, and so should be limited as much as possible. Here's a list of how much caffeine there is in a five-ounce cup of coffee and a five-ounce cup of tea:

COFFEE (5 ounces)	CAFFEINE
Drip	110–150 mg
Percolated	64–124 mg
Instant	40–108 mg
Decaf	2–5 mg
Instant Decaf	2 mg

TEA (5 ounces)	
One-minute brew	9–33 mg
Three-minute brew	20–46 mg
Five-minute brew	20–50 mg
Instant tea (5 ounces)	12–28 mg
Iced tea (12 ounces)	22–36 mg

In 1990, Dr. Robert Heaney and his associates at Creighton University in Nebraska reported the results of a study in which sixteen women were given four 100-mg caffeine tablets a day (a total of 400 mg) for nineteen days. All of the women had calcium intakes of at least 600 mg per day. They also took a multivitamin as a source of vitamin D. They concluded that 400 mg of caffeine per day was apparently not harmful, if the women were also getting at least 600 mg of calcium in their diets each day. They also suggested that the increased loss of calcium in the urine from drinking caffeinated coffee may have occurred only in the first three hours after drinking the coffee, and did not persist for the rest of the day. I suggest to my patients that they try to limit their coffee consumption to two cups a day—that's cups (5 ounces), not mugs (10 ounces). Here's the lowdown on the amount of caffeine in various beverages, according to the U.S. Food and Drug Administration and the National Soft Drink Association:

SOFT DRINKS (12 ounces)	CAFFEINE
Coca-Cola	45.6 mg
Diet Coke	46.5 mg
Pepsi-Cola	38.4 mg
Dr Pepper (diet or regular)	42.0 mg
Mountain Dew	54.0 mg
7-UP	0 mg
Root beer	0 mg
Sprite	0 mg

Caffeine-free Coke
  or Pepsi (diet or regular)   **0 mg**

My feeling is that if you keep your coffee consumption to two cups a day—or, even better, switch to decaf—and you try to limit yourself to no more than one soft drink a day, you should be fine.

LOW CALCIUM AND VITAMIN D

In Chapters 5 and 7, I'll go into great detail on the importance of adequate calcium in your diet and why vitamin D is necessary to make that calcium bio-available (which is a fancy way of saying absorbable). It should be pretty clear by now that it is important to eat lots of green, leafy vegetables and low-fat dairy products like yogurt, cheese, and milk every day, so you can get a jump start on overcoming the calcium deficiency that more than 50% of all Americans have.

LOW BODY WEIGHT

If you are a small-boned, lightweight person, then your risk of developing osteoporosis is particularly high. Several studies suggest that if you weigh less than 127 pounds you are especially susceptible to developing osteoporosis. This has always seemed a little arbitrary to me, since 127 pounds on a petite, five-foot-two-inch woman is considerably different from 127 pounds on a five-foot-eight-inch woman, but whatever the source of this figure, the point is that you can be too thin. Appropriate body weight, as well as weight-bearing exercise, goes a long way toward protecting our bones. If you are underweight for your height and frame, I'd suggest you start doing something about that now. A healthy, calcium-rich diet is just what the doctor ordered.

CERTAIN MEDICATIONS

There are a batch of medications that interfere with calcium absorption, or bone remodeling and formation, thereby leaving the patient more susceptible to developing osteoporosis. This can create a tricky situation, since most of the time these medications are vitally important to a patient's general health. If you are taking one of these medications or are planning to do so, be sure to let your doctor know about your concerns relating to their impact on osteoporosis. As long as you are carefully monitored for signs of weakening bones, everything should be fine. Here are some of the medications to watch out for:

Steroids or Corticosteroids and Adrenal Corticosteroids

These drugs do the work of the adrenal glands, the two small glands about the size of a grape located on top of your kidneys. They produce cortisone-like chemicals that include sex hormones as well as the hormones that convert starchy foods into glucose. They also produce hormones that maintain fluid balance and reduce inflammation. For people with an adrenal deficiency such as Addison's disease, or with lupus or rheumatoid arthritis, long-term use of these corticosteroids can reduce swelling, redness, and pain. They are frequently prescribed to treat asthma, bronchitis, allergic diseases, chronic obstructive pulmonary disease (COPD), eye diseases, rheumatoid arthritis, ulcerative colitis, arthritis, psoriasis, lupus, Crohn's disease, multiple sclerosis, some skin diseases, and some types of cancer. When used for a short time or injected into a joint or swollen area there is no effect on bone health, but when used for long periods of time they start to destroy the bone-building process and enhance the process of bone breaking down. Some of the more frequently prescribed steroid drugs are prednisone, prednisolone, Medrol, Deltasone, Decadron, cortisone, Cortel, Celestone, and Aristocort.

Thyroid Medication

The thyroid is a powerful gland located on the front lower part of the neck. Among other things, it regulates metabolism. When the thyroid is over-stimulated, we develop what is called *hyperthyroidism*. When it is under-stimulated, we get *hypothyroidism*. Long-term use of medications to control the activity of your thyroid can interfere with bone health.

Antacids with Aluminum

These medications are used to treat heartburn, indigestion, excess stomach acid, ulcers, and gastric reflux disease, as well as a calcium supplement. Some of these antacids are salts derived from mineral sources, including aluminum. The aluminum is the problem when it comes to bones. When you take an aluminum-based antacid, your body is unable to absorb the calcium and phosphate it needs, and so you increase your risk factor for osteoporosis. Taking an occasional aluminum-based antacid is fine, but if you use them every day they can harm bones. Non-aluminum-based antacids do not deplete bone, so you can take them as often as you'd like.

Here are a few of the more popular aluminum-based antacids on the market: Aludros, Amphojel, Gaviscon, Gelusil, Kolantyl, Maalox, Mylanta, Riopan.

And here are some non-aluminum-based antacids: Alka-Seltzer, Bisodol, Mylicon, Rolaids*, Titralac,* and Tums*. The antacids with an asterisk (*) contain calcium carbonate, which is a supplement beneficial to bones.

Anticonvulsants

Anticonvulsant medication works to prevent seizures by inhibiting the repetitive spread of electrical impulses along nerve pathways. It also has an effect on the liver's ability to metabolize vitamin D. When vitamin D is not properly metabolized, the body is unable to absorb calcium very well. Phenytoin (trade name Dilantin) is the most commonly used anticonvulsant. Phenobarbital is used less often but has the same effect. Since these drugs must be taken for a lifetime, it is important for those who use them to take a calcium and vitamin D supplement.

Diuretics

Diuretics increase the volume of urine. They are used to treat high blood pressure and congestive heart failure by decreasing the blood volume and thereby lightening the workload on the heart. There are several classes of diuretics. The class that is a problem for bone health includes those that are called *loop diuretics,* because they work in an area of the kidney called Henle's loop. Loop diuretics cause the kidney to excrete excess calcium. As a matter of fact, they are so good at doing this, they are often prescribed for people who have too much calcium in their systems. The most popular forms of this drug are Lasix, Aldactone, Dyazide, Bumes, Diamox, and Edecrin. If you take one of these, you need to drink lots of water and add extra calcium to your diet.

Lithium

Lithium, sometimes considered a miracle drug, is used to treat patients with bipolar disorder, a condition often marked by wide mood swings. One of its side effects is the increased production of parathyroid hormone, which in turn increases the breakdown of bone. If you are taking lithium, make sure you keep physically active and get adequate calcium in your diet through food and supplements. Lithium is a benzodizepine, a class of drugs that also includes Valium and Xanax, so be sure to check with your doctor if you are taking one of these.

Heparin and Coumadin

These are blood-thinners or anticoagulants, sometimes administered in the hospital. If you take them for a long period of time, pay close attention to your bone health, get whatever exercise your doctor feels is safe for you, and make sure there is lots of absorbable calcium in your diet.

Antibiotics

Prolonged or frequent use of antibiotics, especially tetracycline, can impair bone health. Be sure to bring this up with your doctor if you have been on antibiotics for an extended period of time.

Methotrexate

This medication is used to treat arthritis, cancer, psoriasis, and immune disorders. It also can cause bone damage, so check with your doctor on what precautions you should take to protect your bones.

It is clear that if you are on any of these medications, you are on them for a reason. It is good to be aware that prolonged use of them can put your bones at risk, so you should discuss this with your doctor. Follow his or her advice, keep moving and eating calcium-rich foods, and you can do a lot to keep your bones healthy, strong, and beautiful.

What Is the Bone Mineral Density (BMD) Test All About?

Now that you know how important it is to get a BMD test if you are at risk for osteoporosis, let me explain what a BMD test is and what kinds there are.

A BMD test is a simple, noninvasive procedure to measure bone density, which is a measure of bone strength. Bone density refers to just how much mineral and trabeculae are contained in a particular amount of bone—for example, how many grams of mineral are in a square centimeter of bone. The more dense your bones, the stronger they are. Regular X rays cannot show subtle loss in bone density. It is true that the stronger your bones in general, the whiter they appear in an X ray, but in terms of the whiteness of the image, an X ray of the spine will not show bone loss until you have lost about 30% of bone density in that area. Sometimes an X ray is used to determine bone density in the hand and forearm, but these X rays are then put into a computer that digitalizes them and analyzes how white they are, and therefore, how dense.

DEXA (sometimes called DXA), or dual-energy X-ray absorptiometry, is considered state-of-the-art in BMD testing today. The FDA approved DEXA testing in 1988. With an X-ray tube containing no radioactive isotope, DEXA can measure the bone density of virtually every area of the skeleton. It is incredibly fast. Whereas some of the earlier methods, called SPA, can take up to twenty-five minutes to measure the density of the spine, a conventional DEXA machine can do it in two to four minutes, and some of the newer models can perform the same test in thirty seconds. DEXA hip study takes between two and four minutes, and the whole body can be studied for bone density in ten minutes. The radiation exposure is minimal—only about ¹⁄₁₀ that of a chest X ray—and the results are highly accurate. Changes in bone density as small as 1–4% per year can now be measured. We can now tell, very precisely, whether a patient's recommended bone therapy is working.

DEXA refers to a technique, not to any particular machine made by a particular manufacturer. A central DEXA device or tabletop machine is the name usually given to the machines that measure the spine and hip, though these machines can also measure bone density in the wrist, heel, or total body. The procedure with any of the BMD measuring devices is completely painless, noninvasive, and easy. You simply lie down on the large DEXA machines as you would for an X ray, but you can keep all your clothes on. In just a few minutes you are up and ready to go. Some of the other measuring devices are:

SEXA, the X-ray Version of SPA

Single-energy X-ray absorptiometry is the X-ray replacement for the older SPA devices, which used radioactive iodine to measure bone density. These machines can measure only the wrist and heel, not the spine or hip. Both machines require that the heel be submerged in a gel- or waterlike substance during the test. Both machines have generally been replaced by DEXA machines.

Computerized Axial Tomography

Sometimes referred to as a CAT scan or CT scan, this method can also measure bone density in all parts of the body. CAT of the spine exposes patients to more radiation than does DEXA, but some doctors prefer this method because it actually provides a three-dimensional measurement of the bone. CAT bone measurements are given in milligrams per cubic centimeter, not grams per square centimeter as with DEXA (two-dimensional) measurements. CAT is not used to measure bone density in the hip.

QUS (Quantitative Ultrasound)

Yes, it's true, ultrasound can measure bone density. This method is usually used to measure the heel, but it can also be used to take measurements from the kneecap (patella), from the front of the lower portion of the leg (tibia), and from the fingers. There is no radiation in this test, but it does require the application of gel to the skin. QUS measures the speed at which sound waves pass through the bone and the amount of energy that is lost from the sound wave as it passes through the bone, the broadband ultrasound attenuation (BUA). QUS is just another way of measuring bone density without using X rays.

As I've already explained, the most important number on the bone density test, no matter what method you use, is your T-score. The World Health Organization (WHO) established the T-score criteria in 1994. Because they designed it based on studies of postmenopausal Caucasian women, it is not clear how appropriate it is for other groups, but at the moment it provides the standard that most doctors use. Your bone density is normal if it is not more than one standard deviation below the average for a young adult. You have osteopenia if your T-score is between –1 (minus one) and –2.5 (minus two point five). You have osteoporosis if your T-score is below –2.5 (minus two point five).

It is true that you can break a bone even if your bone density is perfectly normal, depending on the severity of impact. If you have osteopenia, however, your risk factor for breaking a bone goes up, and if you have osteoporosis, it goes way up. In fact, the risk factor for having a fracture doubles for each standard deviation decline in bone density. Another way of putting this is that your risk factor doubles each time the T-score goes down by 1.

WHAT DOES THIS HAVE TO DO WITH ME?

There are many ways you can help reduce your risk of getting osteoporosis:

○ Start exercising, today.

○ Quit smoking. I know it is hard, but it is one of the best things you can do for bone health, and for your health in general.

○ Limit your alcohol consumption to two drinks a day.

○ Switch to decaffeinated coffee, or try to limit yourself to two five-ounce cups of coffee and one soda a day.

○ Eat foods high in calcium.

○ If you are a postmenopausal woman, keep your body weight over 127 pounds.

○ If you are on steroid medications, antibiotics for an extended period of time, lithium or other bone-threatening medications, check with your doctor, and increase your calcium intake.

And let me remind you:

○ If you are a Caucasian woman over sixty-five, get a BMD test.

○ If you are a Caucasian woman under sixty-five but have at least one risk factor for osteoporosis, get a BMD test.

○ If you are a man or woman of any age or ethnicity in a high-risk group for osteoporosis, get a BMD test.

If you start taking action right now, you can do a lot to save your beautiful bones, and you might even save your life.

CHAPTER THREE

SEPARATING FACT FROM FICTION

*The Ten Most Important Things You Need to Know
to Prevent Osteoporosis*

B EFORE WE GET into the facts, let's take a quick look at some of the popular fictions that have sprung up on the topic of osteoporosis. The following is a list of what I consider to be the ten most common myths or misconceptions about osteoporosis:

The Ten Most Common Myths about Osteoporosis

Myth #1: Osteoporosis is a little old lady's disease.

Wrong. Rather, right and wrong. Certainly the majority of people with osteoporosis in this country are postmenopausal women—that is, women over fifty-five—but the disease is by no means confined to them. It is a fact that one out of every two postmenopausal women will be affected by osteoporosis. You already knew that. But men develop osteoporosis, too. Actually, one out of every five osteoporosis patients is male, and one out of every three hip fractures occurs in men, although they usually happen at a more advanced age than in women. Then there are the young men and women who have secondary conditions that

---

Life After Menopause

The average American woman lives one third of her life after menopause.

cause them to develop osteoporosis, often because of the medications they are taking. On top of this, there are the young women who have had early menopause, have had their ovaries removed surgically, or have developed amenorrhea (their periods have stopped) from overexercise or some other reason, putting them at high risk for osteoporosis. As I've mentioned before, after the age of about seventy a man's risk of developing osteoporosis is just as high as a woman's, so although older women are the prime candidates for this disease—especially in the first five years after menopause—they are by no means its only victims.

Myth #2: Osteoporosis never killed anybody.

Wrong. As sorry as I am to have to tell you this, osteoporosis can and often does cause premature death. I must emphasize the seriousness of this disease, and I strongly encourage you to do something about it now, while you still can. Every year more than 300,000 people fracture their hips because of osteoporosis. The startling statistic is this: For people over fifty who have osteoporosis and fracture their hip, almost one in four (24%) will die within a year of the fracture, most within the first six months. An additional 25% will require long-term care after the fracture. This means that 72,000 Americans die each year from an osteoporosis-related hip fracture, and an additional 75,000 require long-term care following the fracture. Another statistic that I find shocking is that more than twice as many Americans die from complications resulting from hip fractures than from car accident fatalities each year. There is a reason that this disease is so often called "the silent killer." Just take a look at how osteoporosis-related deaths from hip fracture fit in with the National Center for Health Statistics findings on

> **Osteoporosis Fact**
>
> Osteoporosis can strike at any age in an adult life.

> **Hip-Fracture Statistic**
>
> Approximately 85% of people who fracture their hip do not regain the same mobility and freedom they had before the accident.

the leading causes of premature death in this country in the year 2000. Although no figure is given for deaths from osteoporosis-related hip fractures, I suspect this figure is incorporated into the accidental death figure.

Ten Leading Causes of Premature Death in the U.S.	
1. Heart disease	710,760
2. Cancer (all kinds)	553,091
3. Stroke	167,661
4. Chronic obstructive pulmonary disease	122,009
5. Accidents (all kinds)	997,900
6. Diabetes	69,301
7. Pneumonia and flu	65,313
8. Alzheimer's	49,558
9. Nephritis	37,251
10. Septicemia	31,224

Myth #3: Osteoporosis is a normal part of aging.

Wrong again. It is true that the predisposition for developing osteoporosis increases as we get older, but as I keep reminding you, it is usually preventable and always treatable, though it is not curable. The trick is to try to develop maximum bone mass when we are young, by making sure we have a calcium-rich diet and by staying physically active. But even if we haven't done that, we can still reduce our risk of developing osteoporosis as adults by doing the same thing now: eating lots of calcium-rich foods and engaging in a regular exercise program. If you should fall into any of the high-risk categories, it is important to get a bone density test so that if your doctor detects the beginning of a problem, he or she can prescribe the appropriate medication to treat it before it has a chance to develop into osteoporosis. Prevention is always the best cure in any branch of medicine, and this is particularly true when it comes to osteoporosis, since it is so easy to prevent.

Myth #4: I've already been diagnosed with osteoporosis, so there is not much I can do about it.

Absolutely ridiculous! If you have been diagnosed with osteoporosis, you should be talking to your doctor to find out how advanced your condition is and just what the best course of action might be. Any well-informed medical practitioner will tell you that there are many highly effective, FDA-approved medications on the market that can help you enormously. Your doctor can tell you which one is likely to be the most effective for your particular needs, and then prescribe the medication for you. I'll be discussing these medications in detail in the next few chapters. However, although these medications are helpful, it is still important to enjoy a diet rich in high-calcium foods, which we'll get to in Chapter 9, and to follow my simple exercise program, which I discuss in Chapter 11. If you have already been diagnosed with osteoporosis, don't waste a minute before beginning to fall-proof your home, in order to reduce the risk of falling down and breaking a bone. Here are some of the most important things to keep in mind:

How to Fall-Proof Your Home

1. Make sure all **railings and banisters** are securely fastened.
2. Make sure all carpeting is secure, and **get rid of throw rugs** altogether.
3. Keep the **floors clear.**
4. **Fasten all electrical cords and cables** to the wall so that you won't trip over them.
5. Make sure all rooms are **well-lit,** so that you can see where you are going.
6. **Arrange furniture** so that you can move around easily, and **eliminate any unnecessary tables, chairs, and clutter.**
7. Install **grab-rails** near the tub and toilet. Use a **toilet seat riser, nonskid mats,** and **adhesive strips** on surfaces that may get wet.
8. Keep the things you use frequently on **lower shelves** so you don't have to reach for them.
9. Install **night-lights** in the **bedroom, bathroom,** and the **hall** between them.
10. **Carry a cordless phone** with you so you won't trip over phone cords or have to hurry to answer a call.
11. Apply **brightly colored adhesive tape** to the outer edge of stairs to make them more visible.
12. Avoid using high-gloss wax on floors, and slippery floors in general.

Since falling presents such a serious danger to people with osteoporosis, it is important to do everything possible to keep from falling. Incidentally, most falls happen to women, in their homes, in the afternoon, according to a 1991 article in the *Annals of Internal Medicine*. Here are a few ways to reduce your risk of falling and breaking a bone:

How to Fall-Proof Yourself

1. Always wear comfortable, low-heeled, rubber-soled shoes.
2. Wear comfortable, nonrestricting clothes.
3. Carry a cane or walking stick.
4. Carry a shoulder bag, backpack, or fanny pack to keep your hands free.
5. Wear short, loose nightclothes that don't interfere with walking.
6. Try to stay home in snowy, icy, or rainy weather. If you must go out, consider using a walker.
7. Wear warm, rubber-soled boots in winter.
8. Try to improve your balance with a few simple exercises (see Chapter 11).

Myth #5: I'm under forty, much too young to worry about osteoporosis.

Nope. It is true that you may be too young to be in a high-risk group for osteoporosis, but certainly there are diseases, medications, and family history that could predispose you to developing osteoporosis, as we've already discussed in Chapter 2. It is important to remember that it is never too early to start taking preventive measures. Eat lots of calcium-rich foods, follow a reasonable exercise routine, stay active, alert, and upbeat, and you will certainly reduce the risk of developing osteoporosis. Did you know that depression in people of any age increases their risk of developing osteoporosis? If you are feeling depressed, do something about it. See a doctor or psychiatrist or psychologist who can help you talk through your problems, and prescribe appropriate medication if necessary. You may be improving more than your frame of mind.

Another interesting fact is that young women can sometimes exercise too much. You have probably read about some of the female runners and other female athletes who engage in so much physical exercise that their periods stop. This condition is called amenorrhea, and it makes these young women highly susceptible to osteoporosis. Most exercise is extremely good for us, but as with almost anything, when taken to the extreme it can become unhealthy. Finally young people with the eating disorder anorexia nervosa are also at high risk of developing osteoporosis. Anorexia (and bulimia) are most common in young women, and because of the malnutrition and estrogen deficiency that go along with these diseases, it is not uncommon for young anorexic and bulimic women to suffer spinal and other fractures.

Myth #6: Since I'm a man, I have nothing to worry about.

Not at all true! As I've mentioned, one in eight men will develop osteoporosis in his lifetime, and after the age of seventy the risk of developing this "silent killer" is the same in men as it is in women. In fact, a man's risk of developing an osteoporatic hip fracture in his lifetime is about 17%. In men, this type of hip fracture is even more likely to lead to premature death than in women. It is true that women can lose as much as 47% of bone density from their spine and 39% from their wrist in their lifetime, whereas men, on average, lose only 14% from both. This is because in their twenties, men tend to have achieved higher bone density in the first place, and they also tend to be more physically active and less calcium deficient than women. Men who have had the mumps (which can infect the testicles, thereby reducing the production of testosterone) are more susceptible to osteoporosis, and they often incur spine and hip fractures. Pituitary tumors and alcoholism can also cause lowered testosterone levels, thereby leaving a man more vulnerable to osteoporosis.

Not long ago, a strong, healthy-looking forty-two-year-old man came to my office complaining of back pain. I did a routine workup, took some X rays of the spine, and found to my surprise that he had severe osteoporosis. His back pain was probably not related to the osteoporosis itself, but was due to a small, herniated disk. A workup for osteoporosis revealed no abnormal underlying medical conditions. However, his diet was deficient in calcium and his alcohol intake was somewhat excessive. I treated him by altering his diet to include high levels of calcium, vitamin D, and

Men and Hips

Each year about 80,000 men have a hip injury. Men are more likely than women to die within the first year of having a fractured hip.

Elderly Men and Hips

Elderly men account for almost 35% of hip fractures.

Leading Risk Factors in Men

1. Testosterone deficiency
2. Caucasian ancestry
3. Alcoholism
4. Sedentary lifestyle
5. Calcium deficiency
6. Cortisone and other medications
7. Cigarette smoking
8. Lean body build
9. Some gastrointestinal surgery
10. Mumps and other diseases leading to secondary osteoporosis

magnesium and multivitamin supplements, and I prescribed Fosamax. In addition, I started him on an exercise program and got him to limit his alcohol consumption to four ounces of wine a day. One year later, his bone density had improved significantly. A study by the Mayo Clinic found that cigarette smoking and alcohol consumption greatly increase the risk of osteoporosis in men. It is also true that all of the diseases and medications that contribute to osteoporosis in women work the same way for men. Most experts agree that men over fifty should consume 1,500 mg of calcium and 600 to 800 mg of vitamin D a day. If they smoke or drink in excess, they should make every effort to stop or at least cut down. Men should also report any significant loss of sex drive or function to a doctor, since this could be a sign of dipping testosterone levels, which, if not treated, could greatly increase their risk of developing osteoporosis.

Myth #7: If I eat more calcium-rich foods and take a supplement, I'll be just fine.

Not by itself, I'm sorry to say. As marvelous as calcium is for our bones and teeth, it is not a reclusive mineral—that is, it does not work in isolation. It must be accompanied by vitamin D in order to do its job. It is the vitamin D that makes the calcium absorbable, or bio-available, if you prefer the fancy word. Calcium alone has never been shown to improve bone density, but when combined with vitamin D, bone density improves dramatically, and there can be a 50% reduction in the rate of bone fractures. We also need a batch of other vitamins and minerals, including vitamin K (especially helpful for women no longer on hormone therapy), vitamin C, magnesium, boron, potassium and a few others that I will discuss in detail in Chapter 7. Please don't misunderstand me. Of course it is important to get at least 1,500 mg of calcium into our diet each day, but we also need 400 to 800 mg of vitamin D along with these other vitamins and minerals to help our bodies make the most out of the additional calcium it is getting.

Myth #8: Now that I'm no longer on hormone replacement therapy, I'll probably get osteoporosis.

Of course this is not true, and it is just this kind of fear, expressed to me by so many of my patients, that inspired me to write this book in the first place. There is no question that HRT does help protect bone health in postmenopausal women. There is also no question that there are many other ways for postmenopausal women—and everyone else—to protect their bones. A diet rich in calcium and vitamin D, a reasonable amount of weight-bearing exercise, and an awareness of your risk factors are the keys to preventing osteoporosis. As I'll discuss in Chapter 4, there are medications that mimic the effect of estrogen that you can safely take if you feel you need them and your doctor agrees. These drugs are called SERMs—selective estrogen receptor modulators. They work by attaching themselves to estrogen receptors on various tissues, and they produce mild, estrogen-like effects. They do not, however, appear to stimulate the breast tissue the way estrogen does. SERMs are sometimes referred to as "weak estrogens" or "designer estrogens" and they appear to be free of the risky side effects found in more conventional replacement therapies. The first SERM for treating osteoporosis was approved by the FDA in 1998. It is called raloxifene, and it is sold under the trade name Evista. Although it does not reduce hot flashes, it does lower cholesterol—though not as much as conventional HRT—and as I said, it also seems to reduce the risk of breast cancer. It does, however, slightly increase the risk of blood clots. Several other SERMs are being studied right now, and these should be approved by the FDA within the next few years.

Myth #9: Since my mother didn't have osteoporosis, I won't either.

Not necessarily. It is true that if there is osteoporosis in your immediate family, your risk of developing it is greater than if this were not the case, but not having it in the family is certainly no guarantee that you won't get it. You may have several of the other risk factors we have discussed, so try not to be too complacent—stay alert, eat calcium-rich foods, exercise, and get a BMD test if you have one or more of the other risk factors in the quiz on page 26. It is also possible that your mother did have osteoporosis but did not even know it. Because we are much more advanced in our ability to diagnose this disease than we were even ten years ago, your mother may not have had obvious symptoms but still may have had osteopenia, or even osteoporosis. Another thing to consider is that you will probably live longer than your mother, increasing your risk as you age. Although there is a definite genetic predisposition toward osteoporosis if someone in your immediate family has it, this does not necessarily mean that you will develop it, and the converse is equally true. Just because no one in your family has the disease, you are not necessarily home free. If you are a heavy drinker, smoker, or had early menopause, for example, your risks increase, so be on the watch for early warning signs, and get a BMD test if you really want to put your mind at ease.

Myth #10: African-American women don't have much to be concerned about when it comes to osteoporosis.

Wrong again. African-American women are at risk of developing osteoporosis as they go through menopause, even though their risk is somewhat less than for Asian and Caucasian women. The risk for Hispanic women falls between these two extremes. Because African-American women usually have higher bone mineral density than white, non-Hispanic women throughout life, they do experience fewer hip fractures. As they age, however, their risk increases until it is about the same as it is for white women. Here are some interesting statistics from the National Institutes of Health's Osteoporosis and Related Bone Disease National Resource Center:

African-American Women and Osteoporosis

- **300,000** African-American women have osteoporosis.
- **80–95% of fractures** in African-American women are due to osteoporosis.
- African-American women are **more likely to die** after a hip fracture than white women.
- As African-American women age, their **risk of hip fracture doubles every seven years.**
- Diseases common to African-American women, such as **lupus and anemia,** are **linked to osteoporosis.**

> • African-American women consume **50% less calcium** than the recommended daily allowance.
> • 75% of African-American women are **lactose-intolerant**.

African-American women—like all women and men, for that matter—should pay close attention to their risk factors for osteoporosis and get a BMD test at the first indication of trouble.

WHAT DOES THIS HAVE TO DO WITH ME?

Just knowing the difference between the facts and the fictions that so often grow up around the subject of osteoporosis can help you determine just how serious your risk factors are.

There is one more thing I'd like to emphasize. Hip fracture is one of the most dangerous side effects of osteoporosis. The World Health Organization predicts a rise in hip fractures from 1.7 million per year worldwide in 1990, to 6.26 million per year worldwide by 2050. One of the truly frightening things about this, as I have previously pointed out, is that most people never fully recover from a hip fracture. In fact, 24% of people who fracture their hip die within the first year following the fracture. In the U.S. alone in 2003, some 350,000 people were hospitalized for hip fracture, and 90% of these fractures were the result of falls. Although it is true that there are things we can do to minimize the risk of hip fracture—such as clearing out our living space, wearing sensible shoes, doing exercises to improve our balance, and even wearing hip protectors if called for—it is much smarter to do everything necessary to prevent and treat this disabling disease before our hips become so vulnerable.

The simple truth is that we are all at risk of developing osteoporosis. It is a major national and global health problem and it is rapidly turning into a worldwide epidemic. The best thing you can do to prevent this disease is to educate yourself about the risks of developing it, eat right, exercise right, and get tested for this "silent thief" before it begins to steal your major asset—your beautiful bones.

CHAPTER FOUR

THE NEW BONE-BUILDING MEDICATIONS

Fosamax, Actonel, Didronel, PTH, and More—
Which Ones Work, Which Ones Don't;
The Risks, the Benefits;
Which Drugs Not to Take Together

I F YOU HAVE already been diagnosed with osteoporosis or osteopenia, or your doctor feels that you should be on medication to prevent the development of osteoporosis, the goods news is that there are a variety of tested and FDA-approved medications for you to choose from. As recently as the early 1980s, estrogen was the only approved treatment for osteoporosis. Then, in 1985, calcitonin, a bone-preserving hormone, was approved, but the catch was that it had to be taken by injection. It was not until the mid-1990s that things really began to change. The first nonhormonal treatment for osteoporosis, alendronate (Fosamax), was approved by the FDA in 1995, and a few years later raloxifene (Evista) received government approval. Patients today have many more medication choices than ever before, and several promising studies that may provide newer and even more effective treatment. I'll talk about some of this research at the end of this chapter, but for now I'd like to discuss some of the medical options currently available and help you determine which may work the best for you. Just remember, though, that even if you are on a special medication to prevent the advancement of osteoporosis, it is still vitally important to get enough calcium and vitamin D into your diet, through foods or supplements, and to follow a regular exercise program.

The medications we're going to discuss can be extremely important to high-risk patients, but they do not replace nature's natural cures—exercise, calcium, and vitamin D. They simply help them out.

The drugs now available for treating osteoporosis fall into four categories: 1) bisphosphonates (alendronate and risedronate sodium); 2) selective estrogen receptor modulators (raloxifene hydrochloride), referred to as SERMs; 3) calcitonin; and 4) estrogens, which we will discuss, although since the findings of the WHI study, I usually don't recommend estrogens to my patients; and 5) parathyroid hormones. These osteoporosis drugs have been shown to reduce bone loss—in some cases, promote bone growth—cut down on the risk of fractures, and sometimes even ease the pain caused by fractures.

Deciding which drug is best for you will depend on several things, including your gender, age, risk factors, and whether you already have osteoporosis (and how severe it is), or whether you are just trying to prevent the disease. But before starting any drug, consult your doctor. I'll give you a quick breakdown of the pros and cons of each drug before going into a more complete discussion. Let's start with the most popular bisphosphonates: alendronate and risedronate sodium.

BISPHOSPHONATES

Alendronate (Fosamax), Risedronate Sodium (Actonel),
and Etidronate (Didronel)

Alendronate	
Brand name	Fosamax (bone resorption inhibitor) (Merck)
Dosage	For osteoporosis **prevention: 5 mg per day** or **35 mg per week** in a single dose (the preferred method)
	For osteoporosis **treatment: 10 mg per day** or **70 mg per week** in a single dose (the preferred method)
How to take	Take in the morning with an 8-oz. glass of water. Sit upright or stand for thirty minutes after taking, and don't eat or drink anything else during this time. It is only effective on an

	empty stomach. Failure to take as directed can result in inflammation or bleeding ulcers in the esophagus.
Side Effects	Occasional nausea, heartburn, abdominal or stomach pain, difficulty swallowing, bloating, vomiting, constipation, diarrhea and gas.
Cautions	Be sure to let your doctor know if you are taking aspirin or aspirin products, or if you have ever had ulcers, heartburn, stomach, kidney, or esophagus problems.

Bisphosphonates work only on the bone and do not affect the heart, breast, or uterus or other parts of the body. Do not take Fosamax with tea, coffee, juice, or mineral water. Use only eight ounces of natural water, and be sure not to eat or drink anything else for thirty minutes after taking the drug, because this can interfere with the absorption and effectiveness of the drug. If you can wait an hour after taking the drug before eating or drinking anything else, that's even better. Taking nonsteroidal anti-inflammatory drugs (NSAIDs), including aspirin, along with Fosamax can irritate the stomach or intestine, so let your doctor know about it.

Do not take Fosamax if you are pregnant or nursing. It may pose a risk to the fetus. This drug is primarily for postmenopausal women, as well as some high-risk men who are being treated for osteoporosis that has resulted from long-term use of steroid medications such as cortisone and prednisone. Fosamax was the first nonhormonal treatment for osteoporosis. Clinical studies have shown that alendronate prevents bone loss and reduces the risk of all osteoporosis-related fractures, including fractures of the spine and hip in people with osteoporosis.

Who Should Take Fosamax?

This is the drug I most often prescribe for my high-risk patients. It also has been shown to help prevent bone loss in those who decide to go off hormone therapy. A 1999 Spanish study of 144 women who went off HRT showed that after one year, those taking alendronate maintained bone density in their hips and increased bone density in their spines by 2.3%. The women taking the placebo lost 1.4% bone density in their hips and 3.2% in their spines.

Risedronate Sodium	
Brand name	Actonel (Procter & Gamble, Aventis)
Dosage	For osteoporosis **treatment** or **prevention: 5 mg per day or 35 mg per week** in a single dose
How to take	Follow instructions for Fosamax
Side effects	Usually none
Cautions	As with **Fosamax,** let your doctor know if you are taking **aspirin** or aspirin-containing medications, or if you have had any problems with your kidneys, stomach, or esophagus.

This is a newer bisphosphonate. It is much like Fosamax and should be taken just the same way—on an empty stomach, with eight ounces of water. You should remain in an upright position for at least a half hour after taking it, and eat and drink nothing else during that half hour. Research has shown that risedronate sodium can:

- Increase bone mass
- Stop bone loss
- Produce healthy bone
- Reduce spine and hip fractures by 40 to 50% in three to five years
- Decrease risk of vertebral fractures within one year

Although risedronate appears to have a profile similar to that of alendronate, there is some evidence that risedronate may have lower gastrointestinal (G.I.) irritation. A dose of 5 mg risedronate provides only 80% of the hip protection of the 10-mg dose of alendronate, yet the cost is about the same.

Bisphosphonates were originally used only to treat osteoporosis. Now they have been approved as a method to prevent osteoporosis, in a lower dose and in combination with calcium and vitamin D supplements. They are often prescribed for prevention in postmenopausal women and in patients who have steroid-induced osteoporosis. Now that bisphosphonates can be taken just as effectively once a week as they can be every day, my patients find it much easier to comply with the restrictions on how to take them. Some recent studies have suggested that there may not be as many gastric problems associated with these drugs as was originally thought, but the warning on the label about how to take the drug still applies, and I urge you to carefully follow the suggestions on the label.

Another bisphosphonate, etidronate (Didronel), is not prescribed much anymore. It was usually taken once a day for two weeks out of a three-month period, along with calcium every day. It was to be taken two hours before or after meals and separate from other medications such as calcium and vitamins. It was originally developed to treat bone disease and bone cancer, and for a long time it was the only way to treat osteoporosis. The problem is that while it did prevent bone loss by slowing the breakdown of old bone, the bone that was preserved was considerably damaged. Etidronate interferes with the formation of new bone, so that people who took this drug found that although their bones were denser, they were becoming more brittle, which put them at an increasing risk of fracture. Studies have shown that the positive effects of this drug tend to wear off after about two years, and as yet, there are no studies to determine what happens when people take this drug for a long period of time. Since it does tend to create soft bones (osteomalacia) over a period of time, and since several new and more effective drugs are now on the market, etidronate is rarely prescribed anymore, and I do not recommend it.

Unfortunately, some people, though not many in my experience, cannot tolerate oral bisphosphonates. Two bisphosphonates are given intravenously, and these are used for such patients: pamidronate and zoledronic acid (Zometa), made by Novartis. Preliminary results with Zometa suggest that an annual injection can provide the same protection against osteoporosis as taking a smaller oral dose of a bisphosphonate every day.

RALOXIFENE HYDROCHLORIDE (EVISTA)

This class of drugs, called selective estrogen receptor modulators (SERMs), and sometimes refered to as "designer estrogens," are actually not hormones, but they act like hormones in many ways. Raloxifene was approved by the FDA in 1997 to prevent but not treat osteoporosis. Recent studies have shown that it also builds up bone, so it is now approved not only for the prevention but also for the treatment of osteoporosis in postmenopausal women. Incidentally it is the only approved SERM for preventing osteoporosis.

Raloxifene has been shown to:

O Reduce the risk of fractures of the vertebra by 40% to 50%, although it has no apparent protective effect on the hip

O Possibly reduce the risk of breast cancer by as much as 50% over four years

O Decrease total and LDL cholesterol, although it doesn't raise HDL cholesterol

Hot flashes may occur in about 20% of the women taking raloxifene, and there is an associated risk of phlebitis when compared to estrogen. It also may cause leg cramps and blood clots in the legs and lungs. A major study is going on right now to determine what effect, if any, the drug has on the heart, hip, and other organs of the body. Because it apparently does not protect the hip (as far as we know right now), it is considered inferior to the bisphosphonates and parathyroid hormone in treating osteoporosis.

Raloxifene Hydrochloride	
Brand name	Evista (Lilly & Co.)
Dosage	60 mg per day in a single dose
How to take	No restrictions
Side effects	Hot flashes, leg cramps, blood clots

Cautions	**Do not use this drug before menopause. Tell your doctor if you are pregnant or have had a history of blood clots.**

In a recent study of 5,386 women with osteoporosis, those taking the highest doses of the drug (120 mg a day), when compared with women taking a placebo were:

- One third less likely to experience cognitive impairment (trouble with memory, judgment or perception)

- Half as likely to develop Alzheimer's

Further study is necessary to determine if this drug or other SERMs would have the same effect on men, and there are other studies that do not support the correlation between estrogen itself and a reduced incidence of Alzheimer's. Tamoxifen is a SERM prescribed to reduce the recurrence of breast cancer. It also appears to have estrogen-like activity for maintaining bone, but as yet, the FDA has not approved it for the treatment or prevention of osteoporosis.

ESTROGENS

I will mention estrogens here just to be complete in my list of FDA-approved drugs for the prevention and treatment of osteoporosis. As we have discussed, whether or not to take them is up to each woman and her doctor, but since the WHI study results published in July 2002, I usually do not recommend them. Estrogen comes in patches and pills. All estrogen and estrogen-progesterone combination products have been approved by the FDA to prevent osteoporosis, but only some have been approved to treat it.
   Estrogen products include:

- Conjugated equine estrogen, 0.625 mg (Premarin)

- Esterified estrogens, 0.3 mg, 0.625 mg, and 2.5 mg (Estratab)

- Estradiol (Estrace)

- O   Estropipate (Ortho-Est)

- O   Transdermal estrogen patch (Vivelle)

- O   Transdermal estradiol (Climara)

- O   17 beta-estradiol transdermal patches, 0.05 mg (Estraderm)

- O   Piperazine estrone sulfate, 0.75 mg (Ogen)

The estrogen-progesterone products include:

- O   Conjugated estrogen with medroxyprogesterone (FemHRT, Prem-phase, and Prempro)

- O   Estradiol and norethindrone acetate (Activella)

There are several pills, patches, and creams on the market that claim to be "natural" and can be purchased without a prescription. There is no empirical evidence that shows that any of these products provide any benefit at all when it comes to bone loss.

If you have been on HRT and have decided to stop taking it, talk to your doctor about the best way to do that. It is usually recommended that you cut down the dosage gradually over a period of a few weeks, rather than stopping all at once. If menopausal symptoms return, ask your doctor how to best treat them.

CALCITONIN

Calcitonin is a hormone produced by the cells adjacent to thyroid glands of mammals and fish. Synthetic forms have been made from the hormones of humans, pigs, salmon, and eels. It is actually a peptide composed of thirty-two amino acids which bind to osteoclasts and thus inhibit bone resorption. Traditionally, it has been used to treat high levels of calcium in the blood (hypercalcemia), which can happen when someone has cancer, and Paget's disease (a bone disease), as well as osteoporosis in women five or more years after menopause. It can decrease bone loss in the spine, but it is the least potent of all the approved medications. Two studies, using a combined total of 325 women five years after menopause with severe osteoporosis, have shown that calcitonin nasal spray (Miacalcin), increased bone density in the vertebrae by 2% to 3% when compared with women using a placebo (a nasal spray without calcitonin). There was, however, no evidence of this bone-building effect in the hip or forearm of the women in this study.

For maximum benefit, this drug should be taken in combination with calcium and vitamin D supplements. The manufacturer of the nasal spray is conducting a five-year test to see if calcitonin has any effectiveness in reducing the risk of fracture in women with osteoporosis, but the findings of the study have yet to be released. It is also available by injection under the brand name of Calcimar. The bio-availability of nasal salmon calcium is only about 25% of that of intramuscular calcitonin. This means that the biological effect of 50 IU (international units) of intramuscular salmon calcitonin is equivalent to that of 200 IU of nasal salmon calcitonin, but the catch is that the injection often causes nausea, vomiting, and flushing, and these side effects are much less common in the nasal spray. Some studies suggest that calcitonin reduces the pain of acute spinal fractures, although it is not clear why this happens. One theory is that calcitonin causes a rise in endorphin levels. Unpleasant side effects from the nasal spray include runny nose and sometimes even nasal bleeding. If you are using this drug and this happens, call your doctor right away.

Calcitonin is usually not recommended as a first-line therapy because it is expensive (the cost to the pharmacist for 200 IU per day of nasal calcitonin for one month is about fifty dollars), it produces frequent negative side effects, and there is some concern that the patient will develop a resistance to the drug over time.

THE NEWEST GAME IN TOWN: PARATHYROID HORMONE (FORTEO)

This drug, approved by the FDA in November 2002, is the first osteoporosis drug to actually build bone throughout the body. It is a parathyroid hormone (PTH) and is produced by four little pea-sized parathyroid glands that are located near the thyroid gland, but have nothing to do with it. The purpose of the parathyroid glands is to keep the calcium, magnesium, and phosphate levels in our bloodstream just right. In the process of doing this, PTH also controls just how much calcium is in the bone. PTH works by increasing both bone formation by the osteoblasts and bone resorption (elimination) by the osteoclasts. It thickens the trabeculae and increases the thickness of cortical bone so that the bone becomes stronger and less likely to fracture. In contrast to the other medications that mostly slow down bone resorption (loss), PTH actually builds new bone. This represents a major breakthrough for the treatment of severe osteoporosis in both men and women at high risk of fracture. However, too much can leach

The Medical Breakthrough

Teriparatide (Forteo) actually stimulates the number and action of osteoblasts to build new bone. Other medications simply slow the breakdown of old bone.

out calcium from bone, causing severe osteoporosis. A synthetic form of this PTH is called teriparatide, which is sold under the trade name of Forteo and manufactured by Lilly & Co. It requires a daily, self-administered injection into the thigh or abdomen, and it comes with a disposable penlike device that provides twenty doses. Because it is a small protein known as a "peptide," it cannot be taken in pill form, because your digestive system would break it down before it had a chance to reach your bloodstream. Since other osteoporosis drugs are not peptides, they can be taken in pill form.

Research has shown that a daily dose of 20 mcg can reduce the risk of spinal fractures by 65% and all other fractures by 53% after ten months of use. This is great news. Because Forteo increases bone mass at all sites, it also significantly decreases the rate of fracture in the spine and hip. What's more, no increase in fracture risk was seen in the eighteen months after treatment ended, and no major negative drug interactions were observed.

This drug is not recommended for children, adolescents, or people with Paget's bone disease. Side effects are not common, but they can include headaches, leg cramps, or dizziness. PTH is recommended for patients with declining bone densities, patients who incur new fractures while taking bisphosphonates, and for premenopausal women with osteoporosis. There is some question about whether patients should continue to take bisphosphonates while taking PTH. The Osteoporosis Center at the Hospital for Special Surgery generally recommends discontinuing bisphosphonates while taking PTH.

In some animal studies, this drug has been shown to increase the risk of malignant bone tumors (osteosarcomas) after long-term use. So far, no evidence of malignant bone tumors has shown up in humans taking the drug, but at present it is recommended that patients limit their use of this drug to two years.

MIRROR, MIRROR ON THE WALL, WHICH WILL BE THE BEST DRUGS OF ALL?

There will be many. Just as there have been tremendous breakthroughs in the treatment of osteoporosis since the 1980s—when HRT was the only FDA-approved drug for osteoporosis—the next ten years promise equal and even more dramatic breakthroughs. Major studies are going on all over the world in an effort to come up with improved treatments for osteoporosis. Some drugs that previously had been prescribed for other conditions appear to have a beneficial effect on bones, and these are being studied right now.

Statins

Drugs that lower cholesterol are known as *statins*. Millions of people take them every day. Recently, doctors have noticed that their postmenopausal patients who are taking statins such as Zocor have fewer osteoporosis-related fractures than their postmenopausal patients not taking the statins. Researches at Erasmus University in the Netherlands found that statins can reduce the risk of fractures. They studied 3,469 men and women who used statins for a year, and found that those taking the drug had half the vertebral fractures of those people who did not. According to the lead author of the study, Mariette Schoofs, "statins appear to increase bone formation." More study is required, but is nice to know that there are some additional positive side effects to our cholesterol-lowering drugs.

Fluoride

It is a fact that in areas where fluoride is used in the water, there is a lower incidence of osteoporosis. One study showed that people who drank fluoridated water had a higher bone density than those who didn't. Again, more study is needed to determine just how important fluoride is to bone health. Fluorides certainly help prevent cavities in your teeth. When taken for osteoporosis, the bone appears denser on X rays, but apparently this bone is not stronger and breaks just as easily as before. The fluoride deposited on bone gives bone a denser appearance but does not increase the strength of the bone.

Non-Loop Diuretics

Loop diuretics are a class of diuretic agents that act by inhibiting reabsorption of sodium and chloride. They can cause bone loss. Hydrochlorothiazide is a common diuretic that is not in the loop category and therefore does not cause bone loss. A recent study showed that over a three-year period, this drug preserves bone density in the hip and spine when compared with people in the study who were taking a placebo. The benefit was small, but significant enough to encourage further studies.

Natural Estrogens

Many estrogens that come from plant sources (phytoestrogens) such as soy, for example, are being studied for their potential benefits in menopausal relief and bone health. One study at the University of Illinois suggested that women on a high-soy diet for six months had a small increase in spinal bone density, but more research is needed to corroborate this finding. For a while, researchers were excited about the potential bone-health benefits of ipriflavone, a synthetic form of isoflavone, which is a protein found in soy. Some early studies indicated that ipriflavone prevented bone loss and possibly increased bone density, but a more recent double-blind study showed ipriflavone to be no more effective than a placebo.

Estren

In October 2002, researchers reported that when tested in mice, a newly identified synthetic hormone called estren is more effective than estrogen in strengthening bone. Unlike estrogen, it does not increase the risk of breast or uterine cancer. As a gender-neutral treatment that does not affect the reproductive tissues, it can be used in both men and women for the treatment of osteoporosis, according to the journal *Science*. This new compound is years away from human testing, but researchers are very interested in it, because it belongs to a new class of drugs that have the potential to work better to prevent and treat osteoporosis and other chronic diseases of aging than any drugs now available.

WHAT DOES THIS HAVE TO DO WITH ME?

What should be clear to you by now is that if you have been diagnosed with osteoporosis or osteopenia, there is a lot you can do to treat and even reverse your condition. Talk to your doctor and find out which of the drugs we have discussed would be most appropriate for you.

Ten years ago, estrogen was the only medication we had for protecting our bones. Now there are many FDA-approved medications that can help stop and even reverse bone loss. And the future looks bright.

Certainly, studies come and go, or are upstaged by new, contradictory studies, and it is important not to jump to conclusions based on a single, small sample or two. What is important, though, is that so much high-level research is going on in the field of bone health. I'm convinced that within the next five or six years, we will see major breakthroughs in the development of medications and treatments to help us keep our bones strong and healthy. In the meantime, though, it is important to—you guessed it—eat well, exercise often, get a BMD test and, if you have a problem, start treating it right away with one of the many fine osteoporosis drugs already on the market.

PART TWO

THE DIETARY SECRETS THAT CAN CHANGE YOUR LIFE

CHAPTER FIVE

THE CALCIUM REVOLUTION

*The Truth About Calcium; Why It Is the Most
Important Mineral in Your Body,
and the Most Difficult to Absorb*

I BELIEVE THAT we are at the beginning of what is going to become a calcium revolution in this country. As you may have gathered by now, I am a big believer in the benefits of calcium for all sorts of reasons. Calcium is the most abundant mineral in our body, yet sadly, people are becoming increasingly deficient in it. The reason calcium is so important is that it influences all of our major organ systems. Just look at what some of our leading doctors, nutritionists, researchers, and health journalists have been saying about calcium lately:

"'Calcium supplements could inhibit colonic cell proliferation in people susceptible to colon cancer and might also prevent cancer in such organs as the breast, prostate, and pancreas,' says Dr. Martin Lupkin of the Strang Cancer Research Laboratory at Rockefeller University in New York."

> Jane E. Brody, *The New York Times*
> October 13, 1998

"The *Journal of the American Medical Association* reported that with 1,500 mg of calcium a day, cell growth in the colon improved toward normal." (This means that cancer was reversed.)

"The Metabolic Bone Center at St. Luke's Hospital in New York believes that a chronic deficiency of calcium is largely responsible for premenstrual syndrome, PMS."

"In 1997 the large federally-financed trial found that a diet containing 1,200 mg of calcium significantly lowered blood pressure in adults."
Reader's Digest
February 1999

" 'Researchers are increasingly finding that the humble mineral calcium plays a major role in warding off major illnesses from high blood pressure to colon cancer. . . . You name the disease and calcium is beginning to have a place there,' says David McCarron, a nephrologist at Oregon Health Sciences University."
U.S. News and World Report
May 3, 1999

The fact that 44 million people in the U.S. today suffer from low bone mass, and that by the year 2020, the number is expected to rise to 61 million, suggests to me that Americans are already in major calcium deficiency crisis. The good news is that calcium deficiency is easily correctable. All you have to do is become convinced of the importance of this mineral to your overall health, and then learn how to increase the amount of absorbable calcium in your diet every day. I plan to show you how to do this in an easy, efficient, and healthy manner, so that you can make sure your bones are getting the calcium they need to stay strong and flexible. An additional benefit of the 14-day Healthy, High-Calcium Diet, which I'll describe in Chapter 9, is that this diet will not only improve your bone health, it will probably help you feel better than you have for a long time. I have also created the 7-day Healthy, High-Calcium Diet for the Lactose-Intolerant, and the 7-day Healthy, High-Calcium Diet for Vegetarians. These diets have been designed to show you how to get at least 1,500 mg of calcium into your diet every day, naturally, through the foods you eat, while keeping the number of calories in your diet under control. One of these healthy diets should be just right for you.

What is calcium, anyway? It is a soft, malleable, silver-white mineral that makes up about 3.6% of the earth's crust. In fact, it is our fifth most abundant element. It is never found by itself in nature, but exists in compounds such as marble, limestone, feldspar, dolomite, apatite, fluorite, gypsum, and garnet. We've known about it in the form of lime (calcium oxide) since ancient times, but it wasn't actually isolated until 1808 by Sir Humphrey Davy. Calcium sulphate (gypsum), known as plaster of paris, is the substance from which plaster casts are made. It was first used by ancient sculptors to make masks, and later by a doctor in Napoleon's army to immobilize fractured limbs. There is some calcium in almost all plant and animal matter. For us humans, it plays an essential role in forming and maintaining healthy bones and teeth. It is, in fact, the most important mineral in our body, as well as the most plentiful. The average woman has just under two pounds of calcium in her body, and the average man has just over two pounds. One fifth of our total bone mass is calcium.

The strength of our bones (85% of it, to be exact) is determined by the calcium phosphate crystals that are deposited in a collagen matrix in the bone. This collagen matrix, referred to as *collagen type 1*, is actually a protein, and it makes up 35% of the volume of our bones. The rest of the volume comes from other bone minerals that are also composed in large part of these calcium phosphate crystals. Simply put, it is the calcium in our bones that gives them their strength.

What Does Calcium Do for Us?

About 98% of the calcium in our body is stored in our bones. Approximately 1% of it is in our teeth, and the other 1% circulates in the bloodstream and rests in other tissues. Calcium is not only essential for bones and teeth, it also:

- Regulates heart rhythm
- Helps blood clot properly
- Maintains proper nerve and muscle function
- May lower blood pressure
- Eases insomnia
- Increases vitality and endurance
- Helps with the intestinal absorption of many important nutrients, including calcium itself
- Keeps cell membranes healthy
- Helps us metabolize fat and, according to a recent report in the *Journal of the American College of Nutrition*, may even help us lose weight
- May *reduce the risk of cancer*, especially breast and colon cancer

These last two findings are quite extraordinary. Recently the *Journal of the American College of Nutrition* reported on a new study that found that the people who had less calcium in their diets were more likely to gain weight than those who were eating high-calcium diets. In fact an additional 300 mg of calcium per day for adults (you get about 300 mg from one eight-ounce glass of milk) was associated with about six pounds less weight. The reason for this, according to the report, is that *increased dietary calcium makes cells less likely to store fat and more likely to burn fat when calorie intake is reduced.* It appears as though too little calcium in the diet leads to decreased fat burning in the cells, and thus increased fat storage. The study goes on to point out that although it is important to get the recommended 1,500 mg of calcium in your diet every day, there is no added benefit from increasing your calcium intake beyond the recommended level.

Calcium Fact

Adults absorb 25 to 50% of dietary calcium. Most is absorbed in the small intestine.

In another recent study, researchers analyzed the diets of preschool children over a three-year period and found that children with a higher intake of calcium had lower body fat than those children with a lower calcium intake.

When people begin a calcium-rich diet, they often not only report feeling better almost immediately, but they start taking off pounds, as well. Although my diet was not designed with weight loss as its primary goal, this seems to be a secondary benefit that many people welcome. Do be careful, though, if you are a postmenopausal woman. Losing weight too quickly after menopause can increase your risk of developing osteoporosis, so always check with your doctor before starting any weight-loss program.

Two major new studies suggest that adequate calcium in your diet may also reduce the risk of certain types of cancer, in particular colon cancer, the fourth most common type of cancer in the world. Doctors at the University of North Carolina gave 1,200 mg of calcium a day to people who had previously had colon polyps removed. This group had 24% fewer recurring polyps than the people who did not increase their calcium intake, according to Dr. Robert Sandler.

In another study, Harvard researchers collected diet and lifestyle data on more than 100,000 men and women taking part in two large-scale health studies. They were looking for a correlation between calcium intake from both food and dietary supplements and the incidence of colon cancer over a period of sixteen years. They found that increasing dietary calcium did not have much effect on colon cancer for the women in the study, but for the men the impact of additional calcium was profound: An increase of at least 700 mg of calcium per day was associated with a 40% lower risk of colon cancer. They found, however, that this was not a "dose-dependent response," meaning that increasing the dosage over 700 mg did not appear to offer any additional protection.

The *Journal of the National Cancer Institute* reported on another study that found that people who ate a diet high in calcium developed 35% fewer cases of some types of colon cancer than people who had lower calcium consumption. Scientists believe that calcium may inhibit the formation of colon cancer by binding with bile acids and fatty acids, both of which can set off abnormal cell growth in the colon. It is possible that other nutrients in calcium-rich foods may be responsible for the reduction in colon cancer, but in this study the use of calcium supplements was associated with a decreased risk, suggesting that it was the calcium itself, not some other dietary factor, that reduced the cancer risk. Apparently, increasing calcium consumption causes the cells that line the colon to change into lower-risk cell types.

There is some new good news for women, too. In yet another recent study, *premenopausal women with high calcium consumption developed breast cancer at a rate almost 30% lower than women who consumed little calcium.* The same effect was not observed, however, in postmenopausal women in this particular study. Further recent research has suggested that a high calcium intake may offer some reduction in the risk of developing ovarian cancer.

"I think that PMS is a signal that a woman is not taking enough calcium, and a marker for future osteoporosis," says endocrinologist Dr. Susan Thys-Jacobs of St. Luke's-Roosevelt Hospital Center in New York. She led the largest study ever conducted on PMS, which divided 500 women into two groups. One group took 1,200 mg of calcium a day, while the other took a placebo. After three menstrual cycles, the calcium-taking group reported a nearly 50% drop in four major PMS symptoms: mood swings, pain, water-retention, and food cravings. The group taking the placebo saw only a 30% drop in these symptoms. "No other drug addresses all these symptoms as effectively," says Dr. Thys-Jacobs. She suspects that two potent hormones that control the movement of calcium in and out of bones work overtime in some women, causing the unpleasant symptoms of PMS.

Doctors are also beginning to suspect a link between low calcium levels and high blood pressure. In 1997 in Argentina, 591 women took 2,000 mg of calcium a day during pregnancy. Their babies had healthy but lower than average blood pressure for seven years after birth, suggesting that calcium taken by a woman during pregnancy may have a profound effect on the blood pressure of the woman's child.

Obviously, these are all preliminary studies, and much more research is needed to confirm their findings, but I am very excited about what this new research is suggesting. What has become absolutely clear to me is that getting adequate calcium into your daily diet is even more important than we had realized, and the time to start paying attention to how to do this is right now.

The tricky thing about getting enough calcium in your diet is that this precious mineral is not easy to absorb. Much of it passes right through your system and is eliminated without ever getting into your bloodstream and on to your vital organs, bones, and teeth. The irony is that the older you get,

Calcium Fact

You can test your calcium supplement by dropping it into a five-ounce glass of white vinegar at room temperature. Stir gently every five minutes or so. If the tablet hasn't dissolved after half an hour, try another brand. If it hasn't dissolved in the vinegar, it probably won't dissolve in your digestive system either. Calcium capsules are often a good alternative to the solid variety.

the more calcium you need, because your bones lose it much faster than they did when you were younger. Also, the older you get, the harder it is for your body to efficiently use the calcium you give it. Therein lies the problem!

HOW MUCH IS ENOUGH?

It is easy to see why calcium is so important to your overall health, but it is shocking to learn that most Americans have a calcium-deficient diet and are getting far less than they need. Most experts agree that the average American over the age of fifty is getting less than half of the calcium he or she needs each day from daily diet and supplements combined. There are two schools of thought on how much calcium is needed at different stages of life. One comes from the government. The official government U.S. Recommended Daily Allowance (U.S. RDA) for calcium is 1,200 mg of calcium a day for everyone under twenty-five and 800 mg for everyone older than that. I think this is conservative, and most of my colleagues and professional nutritionists agree with me. The guidelines provided by the National Institutes of Health seem more reasonable to most of us.

According to the National Institutes of Health, calcium intake in milligrams per day should be as follows:

AGE	CALCIUM
Birth to six months	400 mg
Six months to a year	600 mg
1–10 years	800–1,200 mg
11–24	1,200–1,500 mg
25–50 (men and women)	1,000 mg
51–64 (women on HRT and men)	1,000 mg
51 plus (women not on HRT)	1,500 mg
65 and older (men and women)	1,500 mg

According to the NIH, then, most adults over the age of fifty should be getting 1,500 mg of calcium every day, not the 800 suggested by the U.S. government RDA. When you see food labeling on products in the grocery store, these percentages are almost always based on the more modest calcium requirements established by the government. What this means, for example, is that when you see a cereal box that says that the cereal provides 50% of the U.S. RDA of calcium, it actually provides 50% of the 800 mg of calcium recommended by the government, rather than 50% of the 1,500 mg recommended by the more generally accepted standards of the National Institutes of Health. In other words, if you are a fifty-five-year-old woman not on HRT, or if you are over sixty-five, that cereal is only giving you about 33% of the calcium recommended by the NIH. Do watch out for this, because as I've said, most food labels are based on the lower government standard—not the more generally endorsed standard recommended by the National Institutes of Health.

The problem adults have with calcium is twofold. First, most don't eat enough

Calcium Fact

Mild calcium deficiency symptoms:
- Arm and leg muscle twitching
- Muscle cramps
- Brittle nails
- Insomnia
- Nerve sensitivity
- Palpitations
- Irritability
- Tooth decay

absorbable, calcium-rich foods each day to meet the generally accepted daily minimum requirements, no matter whose recommendations you choose to follow. The fact is that the average American adult is only getting between 200 and 600 mg of calcium a day in his or her diet, instead of the 1,000 to 1,500 mg recommended by the NIH. As I've said, this means that most Americans over fifty are getting less than half the calcium they need each day in the first place. This is truly alarming.

Calcium Tips

1. Calcium supplements are best absorbed in the intestine when taken with food.
2. Take only 500 mg of calcium at a time.
3. Do not take calcium with high-fat food.
4. Do not take calcium supplements with high-fiber foods.
5. Do not take calcium supplements with iron.

Calcium Fact

Severe calcium deficiency symptoms:
- Abnormal heartbeat
- Depression
- Stiffness in joints
- Tingling in hands and feet
- Osteoporosis
- Osteomalacia in adults
- Rickets in children

Second, even though we may think we are eating a diet high in calcium-rich foods, because much of the calcium we do get from food is difficult to absorb, we are probably not getting nearly as much calcium as we think we are from those calcium-abundant foods. One of the primary goals of *Beautiful Bones Without Hormones* is to explain clearly which foods are high in absorbable calcium and how to get enough of those foods in your daily diet, naturally and deliciously. More about this later.

The danger in being calcium deficient is this. The human body is very smart. It wants to keep the amount of calcium in your bloodstream at just the right level so that there will be enough calcium to do all the good things we've been talking about. To do this the body stores calcium in your bones. *When the calcium level in the blood dips just a little, the body knows it has to get more somewhere, so it takes the needed calcium from the "bone bank."* Obviously, if over time your "bone bank" continues to lose more calcium than it is taking in, you're in big trouble. You will be heading for a bone density crisis that will only be reversed when you figure out how to take in more absorbable calcium than you are losing.

But important as calcium is, it can't do its work alone. In order to do its job effectively, it also needs its friends vitamin D, vitamin C, magnesium, vitamin K, and the trace elements boron, silicon, zinc, and copper. We'll talk about these vitamins and minerals in a later chapter, but before we do, let's take a quick look at what our bones are really all about.

THE TRUTH ABOUT BONES

Did you ever wonder what bones actually are, how they are formed, and what they are made of? Our bones are living tissue. We have 206 of them in our body, and they start out, before we are born, as cartilage. By the end of the first trimester of pregnancy, a cartilaginous skeleton has been formed, and then, as the pregnancy progresses, several things start to happen, transforming the skeleton into bone. In the mid-portion of the long bones—called the *diaphysis* or shaft—specialized cells start growing toward the ends of the bone, where they begin to ossify and turn into actual bone. This process is called ossification. At birth, our bones are mostly hard, except for the growth disk of cartilage known as the *physis,* which lies like a plate between the shaft and the end of the bone, called the *epiphysis.* The *physis,* which is known as the growth plate, allows our bones to keep growing until we reach our mid or late teens. Usually, girls stop growing earlier than boys. Growth stops when the *physis* ossifies. Strangely enough, the only parts of our body that continue to grow as we age are our ears and nose!

Before birth, the center of the long bones becomes hollow, making room for the cylinder-shaped marrow cavity. *Compact bone* (cortical bone), which is hard and dense, forms around this cavity in the last trimester of pregnancy. At the ends of these long bones—the arm bones, leg bones, and thigh bones, for example—the cortical bone gets thinner and there is no longer a hollow center. Instead, this area consists of a latticework pattern of crisscrossing bone spicules called *trabecular* bone. Your ribs, pelvis, and vertebrae consist of trabecular bone with a thin outer layer of cortical bone. You might want to look at the illustration of this on page 15 in Chapter 1.

Within this latticework pattern is the bone marrow that makes the red and white blood cells. When we are born, the long bones have red marrow, but as we mature this marrow becomes yellowish and is made up of fat cells, minerals, and connective tissue. Much of the supportive tissue in our body is collagen, which is the most abundant protein we have. Collagen forms the basic structure of cartilage, ligaments, and tendons, as well as bones. Abnormal collagen can lead to weak and brittle bones. Insufficient collagen reduces the amount of tissue upon which calcium can combine, so these bones are weaker. Collagen is a big help in keeping our bones strong, flexible, and less susceptible to breakage.

Since our bones are living tissue, the old bone is constantly being removed and replaced with new bone. I've discussed this before, in Chapter 1, but let me just review it here, briefly. The fact is that over a period of seven years, every bone in our body is completely replaced. This process is called *remodeling*, and you can see an illustration of this process in Chapter 1 on page 8. Remodeling requires a delicate balance between a batch of cells called *osteoclasts*, which clear away the old bone, and *osteoblasts*, which build the new bone. When we are children our bones are built up much faster than they are broken down. As we age, though, the process begins to reverse and, wouldn't you know, we start to lose more bone than we can replace. When this delicate balance is upset, by either increased activity of the osteoclasts (clearers) or decreased activity of the osteoblasts (builders), our bones become thinner, more brittle, and susceptible to fracture. Osteoporosis, then, is the condition in which bones have become much thinner, more porous, and easily broken. As I've said before, the best way to prevent osteoporosis is through a healthy calcium-rich diet and a bone-strengthening exercise program. Now, let's talk about the diet.

> **Diet Tip**
>
> Sprinkle shredded Parmesan cheese on green vegetables and baked potatoes. Try shaved Parmesan on salads, too.

YOU ARE WHAT YOU EAT

Experts generally agree that food is the best source of calcium. Most of us know which foods tend to be high in calcium. Calcium-rich foods include milk and dairy products, yogurt, cheese, and ice cream. Tofu (soy), dark-green leafy vegetables such as collards, kale, turnip greens, and broccoli, as well as soybeans and bok choy, are also high on the list. Other calcium-rich food groups include fish and shellfish—especially oysters, canned salmon with bones, and canned sardines with bones—shrimp, nuts, eggs, and calcium-fortified cereals, breads, and juices.

Dairy products, in general, provide the best natural sources of calcium in our diet. For those who have no problem with allergies, lactose intolerance, or sensitivity to dairy products, the following is a random list of the amount of calcium in milligrams in various dairy products.

Diet Tip

Use blackstrap molasses to sweeten home-baked breads, cereal, and cakes. Each tablespoon contains 172 mg of calcium.

As you can see, yogurt, milk, and cheese are fine sources of high-quality calcium, and for those who have no trouble digesting dairy products, there is nothing better. But a growing number of people in this country are becoming lactose-intolerant. In Chapter 9, I will go into great detail about calcium-rich recipes and menus for those who have trouble with dairy products. Just remember that even if you

Calcium Content of Various Dairy Products in Milligrams

YOGURT		
Plain, nonfat	1 cup	452
Plain, low-fat	1 cup	415
Fruit, low-fat	1 cup	314
Frozen, low-fat or nonfat	1 cup	300
MILK		
Nonfat, dry	1 cup	1,508
Whole, dry	1 cup	1,168
Condensed, sweetened	1 cup	837
Evaporated, nonfat	1 cup	369
Evaporated milk	1 cup	329
Nonfat (skim)	1 cup	300
Whole milk	1 cup	291
Buttermilk	1 cup	285
Chocolate milk	1 cup	280
Sour cream	1 cup	268
Half and half	1 cup	254
Whipping, light	1 cup	166
Whipping, heavy	1 cup	154

CHEESE		
Ricotta, part skim	1 cup	669
Parmesan (fresh)	1 ounce	336
Romano	1 ounce	302
Gruyère	1 ounce	287
Swiss	1 ounce	250
Monterey Jack	1 ounce	212
Edam	1 ounce	207
Cheddar	1 ounce	204
Muenster	1 ounce	203
Gouda	1 ounce	198
American	1 ounce	195
Mozzarella	1 ounce	183
Parmesan (grated)	1 ounce	168
Fontina	1 ounce	156
Blue cheese	1 ounce	150
Feta	1 ounce	140
Cottage, low-fat, 1%	1 ounce	137
Soft cheese	1 ounce	130
Camembert	1 ounce	110
Goat cheese	1 ounce	85
Brie	1 ounce	52

have no trouble digesting dairy foods, there is slightly more calcium in low-fat milk than in regular milk, so when the option is available, I suggest going for the low-fat dairy products. I will also discuss diets and recipes for people who are vegetarians. A number of my patients are becoming vegetarians, and I caution them to make sure they eat a balanced diet every day. I have created my 7-Day Healthy, High-Calcium Vegetarian Diet on page 204 with them—and all vegetarians—in mind.

Diet Tip

Add skim milk instead of water to condensed soups.

When it comes to nondairy foods that are high in calcium, the following list should give you a fairly good overview of which foods are calcium rich and which are not. As I've mentioned, those of you who are lactose-intolerant can find my 7-Day Healthy, High-

The Approximate Calcium Content in Some Nondairy Foods

SEAFOOD

Mackerel (canned, with bones)	3 ounces	260
Oysters	3 ounces	80
Perch	3 ounces	115
Salmon (canned, with bones)	3 ounces	200
Salmon, cooked	3 ounces	130
Sardines (canned, with bones)	3 ounces	340
Shrimp (canned)	3 ounces	95

VEGETABLES

Acorn squash	1 cup	90
Bok choy (cooked)	1 cup	230
Broccoli (cooked)	1 cup	160
Brussels sprouts	1 cup	55
Collard greens	1 cup	350
Kale (cooked)	1 cup	180
Mustard greens	1 cup	160
Okra (cooked)	1 cup	220
Rutabaga (cooked)	1 cup	100
Turnip greens	1 cup	230

NUTS

Almonds	3.5 ounces	266
Brazil nuts	3.5 ounces	176
Hazelnuts	3.5 ounces	188
Peanuts	3.5 ounces	58
Walnuts	3.5 ounces	94

CALCIUM-FORTIFIED BEVERAGES

Orange juice, fortified	8 ounces	350
Grapefruit juice, fortified	8 ounces	400
Mineral water	1 liter	200
Soy milk, fortified	1 cup	160
Rice milk, fortified	1 cup	240

Calcium Diet for the Lactose-Intolerant on page 190.

Your body cannot produce calcium. It is entirely dependent on the calcium consumed in the foods you eat or in dietary supplements. The body makes no distinction between the elemental calcium that comes from the food you eat and dietary supplements that come from pills, but most nutritionists feel that getting calcium naturally from calcium-rich foods is by far the best way to obtain it. As with most things, nature's way is the better way.

Calcium-fortified foods are fairly new on the market, and they provide a great way to get more calcium into your diet. The next time you go to the supermarket, make it a point to seek out calcium-fortified foods, check their labels, decide which ones appeal to you, and add them to your shopping cart. I was interested to learn that, according to the label, one eight-ounce glass of Tropicana calcium-fortified grapefruit juice contains 400 mg of calcium. The same size glass of Tropicana calcium-fortified orange juice has 350 mg of calcium, while the same eight-ounce glass of skim milk has only 302 mg of calcium.

These lists contain just a sampling of those calcium-rich foods that we should make a point of adding to our daily diet. I've selected these particular foods because for the most part, they are extremely calcium rich and can

easily be added to your diet. I'll go into detail on many others in Chapter 8. What I want to emphasize now, though, is that there are many foods that are high in calcium but also contain oxalates. Oxalates interfere with the absorption of calcium. I like to call these foods false friends, because even though they are high in calcium, the oxalates in them make it difficult for us to get much use out of their calcium. Some of these foods are spinach, parsley, chives, asparagus, beets and beet greens, summer squash, dandelion greens, and even peanuts,

cashews, and almonds. The oxalates in these foods bind with the calcium, making it very difficult for the calcium to break down into an absorbable form in our digestive system. It is interesting, though, that oxalates do not affect any of the other foods we may eat at the same time, so it is certainly not necessary to avoid them altogether. Plus, they are rich in many other valuable nutrients. Just be aware that much of the calcium in these foods will stay right there, in the food, and never get into your digestive system and on to your beautiful bones. This means that we cannot count on their calcium content when we are figuring out how much calcium we are getting each day. Here's a tip, though. When you eat the greens that are high in calcium but also contain a lot of oxalates, squeeze lemon juice on them to help break down the oxalic acid. You still won't get the full benefit of their calcium content, but you'll be able to absorb more of it than you would have otherwise.

Absorption, then, is the crucial issue when it comes to getting the maximum benefit from a high-calcium diet. Stomach acid must be present for us to be able to dissolve calcium, and as with so many other things, as we get older we have less healthy acid to help our digestive system. It is interesting to note that the acid in orange juice and grapefruit juice helps with calcium absorption. I will go into all this in more detail in the diet chapter, but for now it is important to know that several things are essential for metabolizing calcium. In addition to hormones and nutrients, the following are essential: magnesium, vitamin D, vitamin K, and zinc.

Magnesium

Magnesium helps regulate bone metabolism. It is crucial to bone health because it:

○ Helps transport calcium in and out of bone

○ Increases the sensitivity of bone tissue to PTH and active vitamin D

○ Regulates the parathyroid gland

○ Activates bone-building osteoblasts

There is strong evidence that magnesium depletion contributes to osteoporosis. In fact, in many cases when calcium intake is sufficient, magnesium supplements may be even more important than calcium supplements. The appropriate calcium to magnesium ratio is 2:1. This means that if you are taking 1,500 mg of calcium each day, you should also be taking 750 mg of magnesium, and this is especially true if you already have osteoporosis. If you have a heart condition or arthritis, you may need even more magnesium, so be sure to ask your doctor what the appropriate calcium/magnesium ratio is for you.

As with all mineral supplements, I believe that *chelated* forms are the best. A chelated mineral is one that has undergone a procedure that involves binding it to an amino acid or carbohydrate so that it becomes easier to absorb. The evidence shows that chelated magnesium citrate and magnesium glycinate are better absorbed and used by the body than inorganic magnesium oxide. Magnesium citrate also helps prevent calcium-stone formation in the kidneys. High single doses of magnesium may cause diarrhea, so it is better to take several smaller doses with food throughout the day.

Food Sources for Magnesium	
Brown rice	Milk and dairy products
Buckwheat	Molasses
Corn	Nuts (almonds, Brazil, cashew)
Dandelion greens	Rye
Dark-green vegetables (spinach and lettuce)	Seeds (pumpkin, sesame, sunflower)
Legumes (soybeans, dried beans, and peas)	Wheat germ and bran
	Whole-grain cereals

Vitamin D

The "sunshine vitamin" is one of *the* most important regulators of calcium. I discuss it in depth in Chapter 6, but let me touch on just a few of the amazing things about vitamin D. It is essential for:

- Enhancing calcium absorption in the intestine

- Decreasing the excretion of calcium in the kidneys

- Keeping blood levels in the range needed to promote bone mineralization

Unlike calcium, which we have to get from the food we eat and supplements, we can manufacture our own vitamin D. Just exposing our body to sunlight for between five and fifteen minutes a day often gives us all the precious vitamin D we need. We can't always count on the sun, though, because often, depending on the season and the climate, we may not be able to get natural sunlight every day. Also, as we get older, it is more difficult for us to process the sunlight we do get, so vitamin D supplements are even more important.

How much is enough? This is an important question, because too much vitamin D can be toxic, as can too much of many vitamins and minerals. At very high doses, side effects such as hypercalcemia (too much calcium in the blood) can develop, and there is, apparently, some risk of developing kidney stones and calcified soft tissue. The current RDA for vitamin D is 200 IU, but this is only a maintenance level, and in my opinion, isn't nearly enough to give you any therapeutic value. Generally the most effective dosage

Food Sources for Vitamin D

Avocado	Fish-liver oils
Bread, fortified	Herring
Butter and margarine	Mackerel
Cheese, fortified	Milk, fortified
Cereals, fortified	Oysters
Egg yolks	Salmon

is between 400 and 800 IU per day. But remember, more is not better, as I've just explained, and can even be dangerous. The best forms of the supplement are vitamin D3 (cholecalciferol) and vitamin D2 (ergocalciferol). The naturally occurring vitamin D3 is usually preferable to D2.

Vitamin K

Once thought only to play a role in blood clotting, vitamin K is now coming into its own as the new bone-building vitamin. We've known about the importance of vitamin D and magnesium for some time now, but only recently have nutritionists and drug companies been focusing on the importance of the K vitamin. Basically, it attracts calcium to the bone and helps keep it there. It shares with collagen the responsibility for the strength of our bone matrix, and without a strong matrix, it wouldn't matter how dense our bones were, because they would be as crumbly as chalk. Vitamin K:

- Helps with the formation of healthy bones
- Helps maintain healthy bones
- Slows and may even stop bone loss
- Speeds up the healing of fractures
- Helps maintain the membranes of our cells
- Is a major influence in blood clotting
- Aids in fat synthesis

Our body also makes its own vitamin K. It is manufactured by bacteria in the small intestine, and because antibiotics can kill those bacteria, many researchers feel that this explains the connection between antibiotic use and damage to our bones. If you have been taking antibiotics for an extended period of time, you might want to discuss this potential problem with your doctor.

It is also interesting to note that a large-scale study of women and nutrition found that women who received more than 100 mcg of vitamin K a day were almost one third less likely to fracture a hip than those who had less vitamin K in their diet. Most important of all our purposes, studies have shown that vitamin K is especially helpful for women who are not on hormone replacement therapy.

The daily dose I recommend is between 100 and 300 mcg—notice that that is micrograms, not milligrams. Like vitamin D, vitamin K can be toxic in doses as low as 50 mg, so take it easy. Also it should not be taken if you are on blood thinners such as Coumadin or warfarin.

Food Sources for Vitamin K

Broccoli	Chickpeas
Brussels sprouts	Scallions (raw)
Cauliflower	Spinach

Zinc

We have about two grams of zinc in our body, and most of it is found in our bone tissue, eyes, liver, and, in males, prostate. Zinc is important because it plays an essential role in DNA and protein synthesis, and it is necessary for the formation of osteoblasts and osteoclasts, meaning it influences the turnover of bone. Researchers consider zinc loss a marker for osteoporosis, because studies show that postmenopausal women often have a significant increase in the loss of zinc, and these are the women most susceptible to developing osteoporosis. Zinc is responsible for:

O Producing both osteoblasts and osteoclasts

O Helping bone to heal

O Helping vitamin D function

O Stimulating the release of hormones

O Metabolizing protein

O Relieving stress

I recommend 12 mg of zinc a day for women, and 15 mg for men, to be taken in its most absorbable chelated forms: zinc glycinate, zinc picolinate, and zinc citrate. There are some foods that inhibit the absorption of zinc. They are brown rice, whole-grain cereals and breads, wheat bran, and legumes (soy beans, dried beans, and peas). Try to take your zinc at meals when you are not eating these foods.

Food Sources of Zinc		
Brazil nuts	Oysters	Pumpkin seeds
Egg yolks	Peanuts	Rye
Meat	Pecans	Split peas
Oats	Poultry	

Healthy bones also require vitamin C, vitamin B6, vitamin B12, folic acid, phosphorus, copper, boron, manganese, silicon, strontium, and selenium, and I'll discuss these in more detail in Chapter 7. For now, here is a list of the vitamins and minerals I suggest you take every day along with the recommended dosage of each. You can get my recommended daily dosage by taking these pills in individual tablets or in multivitamins, but if you decide to take a multivitamin, make sure it does not contain toxic levels of vitamin A, as many do. As I've said, I'll explain in more detail how these and other substances interact to prevent osteoporosis in Chapter 7, but for the moment it is important to start thinking about just how much calcium is in the foods you eat, and how to go about increasing the calcium-rich foods in your diet, each and every day.

Daily Nutrients for Beautiful Bones	
VITAMINS	
Vitamin A (as beta-carotene)	3,000 mcg (or 10,000 IU)
Vitamin C	1,000 mg, divided
Vitamin D	400–800 IU
Vitamin K	100–300 mcg
Vitamin B6	5–25 mg
Vitamin B12	2.4 mcg
Folic acid	400 mcg

MINERALS	
Boron	2–3 mg
Calcium	1,500 mg, divided
Copper	2.5–10 mg
Magnesium	750 mg (2:1 ratio with calcium)
Manganese	3.5–7 mg
Silica	20–30 mg
Zinc	12 mg for women 15 mg for men

Finally, I'd like to talk about the kinds of calcium supplements available on the market today, and which ones I feel work best. The two most popular supplements are calcium citrate and calcium carbonate. Whatever form of calcium supplement you decide to take, remember that it is important to take no more than 500 mg at a time. That is all we are able to absorb at one time, so divide your supplements up and take them throughout the day, always with meals if you are taking calcium carbonate.

Calcium citrate, according to some new studies, may be more easily absorbed than calcium carbonate. It also has the advantage of containing acid, and this helps with absorption. What this means is that you can take calcium citrate with or without food, although most of my patients prefer taking it with a meal. Calcium citrate contains only 200 to 300 mg of elemental calcium per pill, so you may have to take it more frequently than calcium carbonate, and it tends to be slightly more expensive than other calcium supplements. For my money, though, it is the most effective form to take.

Calcium carbonate is the most prevalent type of calcium supplement on the market. It comes in many forms, including pills, capsules, chewable tablets, antacids such as Tums, and caramel chews. Most of these supplements contain between 200 and 500 mg of elemental calcium per pill, but they do not contain acid, so it is important to take them with meals to maximize absorption.

Even though I feel that calcium citrate has a slight edge over calcium carbonate, both forms are fine. See which one best agrees with you and go with it. I would suggest that you choose a brand that also contains 400 IU of vitamin D, since as you know by now, vitamin D helps greatly with absorption. Finally, if you take just one supplement a day, take it in the evening, just before you go to bed, if it is calcium citrate, or after dinner if it is calcium carbonate. Because your digestive system works more slowly at night, the calcium and vitamin D will have more time to get absorbed.

The chart on p. 96 will give you a clear idea of just how much elemental calcium there is in the various commercially available forms of calcium. By elemental calcium I mean the amount of calcium in each tablet that can actually be absorbed by the average person. I'd suggest that you experiment with various brands and dosages until you find one that gives you what you need without upsetting your stomach. Remember, even though you may actually take in 1,500 mg of calcium a day, your body is not going to absorb all of that. As I've said, absorption depends on your age, metabolic rate, activity level, and gender. Just make sure you get 1,500 mg of calcium and do everything we've been talking about to help your body absorb it. Some people find that calcium carbonate can cause gas, bloating, and mild indigestion, while calcium citrate usually has no negative side effects. For most people, though, both forms of calcium supplements are free from negative side effects.

Always check the label on your calcium supplements to see just how much available calcium there is in each tablet. Unfortunately, this isn't always easy to do, because many manufacturers don't make this information clear on the label. If you have trouble figuring out how much calcium is actually available to you in the different name-brand calcium products, just refer to the chart for a precise assessment. By the way, taking a calcium supplement does not mean that you shouldn't also eat lots of calcium-rich foods each day. The pills are more like an insurance policy, just a backup to make sure your bones are getting all the calcium they need.

Many of my patients have been confused about just what elemental calcium is, so let me try to clear this up. Calcium is an element like oxygen, hydrogen, or iron. It cannot be broken down into any other forms. Elements combine with each other to form compounds that are also known as molecules. Calcium combines with the two elements carbon and oxygen to make the common dietary calcium formulation known as calcium carbonate, which incidentally is the main ingredient in Tums and Rolaids. The molecule known as calcium carbonate contains elemental calcium, elemental carbon, and elemental oxygen.

When we digest calcium carbonate, the calcium that was bound to the oxygen and carbon breaks away and returns to its essential form. This substance is known as elemental calcium. The percentage of elemental calcium in calcium carbonate that is available for our bodies to absorb is 40%. This is the number of milligrams of elemental calcium that we need to count toward meeting our daily recommended intake of calcium. Another way of looking at this is that for every tablet that contains 1,000 mg of calcium carbonate, only 400 mg (or 40%) of that amount is available to us for absorption in the form of elemental calcium. The remaining 60% of that tablet is made up of oxygen and carbon.

All calcium supplements work the same way. They contain different amounts of elemental calcium, depending on their particular formulation. Calcium citrate, for example, provides 24% of elemental calcium, though some biochemists argue that it contains as little as 20%. Working with the 24% figure, this means that if you take a 1,000-mg tablet of calcium citrate, only 240 mg of elemental calcium will be available to you. Here is a breakdown of the average actual amount of elemental calcium in the various forms of calcium supplements. Always check the label of the supplement you purchase to see precisely how much elemental calcium it contains.

Calcium Fact

Calcium carbonate
  40% calcium
Calcium citrate
  20–24% calcium
Calcium lactate
  13% calcium
Calcium Sluconate
  9% calcium

Calcium carbonate contains 40% elemental calcium. It is included in supplements such as Os-Cal, Tums, Viactiv, and Caltrate. These supplements are usually derived from oyster-shell powder or limestone rock. They are best taken with meals because they require gastric acid for absorption. Also you shouldn't take more than 500 mg at a time, so consider taking one with breakfast and one with dinner. Some people find that they cause gas and mild indigestion.

Calcium citrate contains 24% elemental calcium. The popular forms of this supplement are Citrical, Citrical with vitamin D, and Centrum for Bone Health. Three new studies reported in the *American Journal of Therapeutics* and the *Journal of Clinical Pharmacology* have concluded that calcium citrate is better absorbed than calcium carbonate by approximately 25%. This is often the preferred supplement for older people who have decreased gastric acid. It need not be taken with meals and usually has no negative side effects, such as gas or bloating.

Amount of Elemental Calcium in Various Supplements

NAME	TYPE OF CALCIUM	ACTUAL CALCIUM AMOUNT
Alkaments	calcium carbonate 850 mg	340 mg per tablet
Biocal	calcium carbonate 625	250 mg per tablet
Biocal	calcium carbonate 1,250	500 mg per tablet
Calcium carbonate, liquid	calcium carbonate 1,250	500 mg per dose
Calcium carbonate tablets	calcium carbonate 500 mg	200 mg per tablet
Calcium gluconate tablets	calcium gluconate 500 mg	45 mg per tablet
Calcium lactate tablets	calcium lactate 650	84.5 mg per tablet
Caltrate 600	calcium carbonate 1,500	600 mg per tablet
Caltrate 600 + D	calcium carbonate 1,500	600 mg per tablet
Digel tablets	calcium carbonate 280	112 mg per tablet
Tums	calcium carbonate 750	300 mg per tablet
Tums Ultra	calcium carbonate 1,000	400 mg per tablet
Citrical + D	calcium citrate 630 mg	151 mg per tablet
Citrical + Magnesium	250 mg	75 mg per tablet

Tribasic calcium phosphate contains 39% elemental calcium. The popular form of this supplement is called Posture.

Dibasic calcium phosphate contains 30% elemental calcium. This is found under the trade names of Shaklee and Dical-D. This calcium attached to phosphate is the naturally occurring calcium found in milk and dairy products.

Calcium lactate contains 18% elemental calcium. This is not a common form of calcium supplement. It is known under the trade name of Shaklee's Calcium Complex, and it also contains calcium carbonate, calcium lactate, and calcium gluconate, along with magnesium, zinc, copper, manganese, and sodium.

Calcium gluconate contains 9% elemental calcium. This also is not a common form of calcium, but it too is known under the trade name Shaklee's Calcium Complex as well as Calcet and Fosfree.

Another way to look at elemental calcium is to consider how many tablets of each supplement you would have to take to actually get 1,000 mg of elemental (absorbable) calcium. Here are a few examples. A calcium carbonate tablet at a strength of 650 mg of calcium (the strength is the number listed on the label) would contain 260 mg of elemental calcium, so you would have to take four tablets to get 1,000 mg of elemental calcium. If the strength of the calcium carbonate tablet were 1,500 mg, it would contain 600 mg of elemental calcium, so you would only have to take two tablets to get 1,000 mg of elemental calcium. A calcium citrate tablet at a strength of 950 mg of calcium would contain 228 mg of elemental calcium, so you would have to take four tablets to get 1,000 mg of absorbable calcium. If, on the other hand, you were to take calcium gluconate at a strength of 650 mg, the amount of elemental calcium would only be 45 mg, so you would have to take a whopping seventeen tablets to get 1,000 mg of elemental calcium into your system.

I usually recommend calcium citrate supplements for my patients, because even though you have to take more of them, the new studies conclude that they are 25% more absorbable than other supplements, and they usually have no unpleasant side effects.

WHAT DOES THIS HAVE TO DO WITH ME?

Calcium is the most important mineral in your body, but most of us are not getting nearly enough of it each day in an absorbable form. If you follow my guidelines for daily vitamin and mineral supplements, and begin to pay attention to getting more highly absorbable, calcium-rich foods into your diet each day, you'll be taking the first, essential steps toward building strong, healthy, beautiful bones.

I'll go into more detail on which specific vitamins and minerals you need, and why, in Chapters 7 and 8, but for now I suggest you try to make sure you are getting at least the following amounts of these important nutrients into your diet each day:

Calcium	**1,500, divided**
(preferably calcium citrate)	(500 mg 3 times per day)
Magnesium	**750 mg**
	(2:1 ratio with calcium)
Vitamin D	**400–800 IU**
	(when you can't get fifteen minutes of sunlight a day)
Vitamin K	**100–300 mcg**
Zinc	**12 mg for women**
	14 mg for men

CHAPTER SIX

LET THE SUN SHINE IN

How Five to Fifteen Minutes of Sunlight a Day Guarantees All the Essential Natural Vitamin D You Need

YOU KNOW HOW GOOD it feels when you walk down the street on a bright, warm spring day and the sun just seems to caress your skin? It turns out that the sun is not just good for your mood and emotional health, it also plays a vitally important part in your physical well-being. The reason for this is that the ultraviolet (UV) rays from the sun trigger vitamin D syntheses in the cholesterol in our skin, and we need this vitamin D in order to absorb calcium and phosphorus, both so necessary for our bones. It is imperative that we get adequate amounts of vitamin D, whether it is through diet, supplements, or by exposing our skin to sunlight for no more than five to fifteen minutes a day, as often as we can. Sometimes, when I see photographs of people sunbathing, it makes me smile, because I remind myself that they are not just lying there doing nothing, they are actually manufacturing something, and that something is vitamin D.

It is important, by the way, to wear no sunscreen or, if you must, a very mild one when you undertake this manufacturing process. Sunscreens with a protection factor (SPF) of 8 or greater will block the UV rays that produce vitamin D. I realize that many dermatologists would be horrified to hear this advice, since too much exposure to the sun can lead to melanoma and other dangerous skin cancers, but since vitamin D is so important in our ability to absorb calcium, and since good calcium absorption is so important in keeping our bones healthy, I always recommend that my patients try to allow their skin (hands, arms, face, and torso) to get just a little natural ex-

Sunlight's Secret

Just fifteen minutes of sunlight a day on fair skin should result in the production of 100 to 200 units of vitamin D3. Darker-skinned people need somewhat longer exposure (perhaps twice as long), since skin pigmentation screens sunlight and reduces the production of vitamin D.

Sunshine and Vitamin D

The fairer your skin, the more vitamin D you make.

posure to sunlight each day. After between five and fifteen minutes, however, it is very important to apply a strong sunscreen (at least 15 SPF), wear a hat, cover up, and limit your time in the direct sun.

Getting a little sun each day is not always so easy. Depending on where you live, the time of year, and how often you are able to get out into the sun, getting enough sunlight to provide you with all the vitamin D you need can be difficult. For example, if you live in Boston or a similar northern climate, the average amount of sunlight from November through February is insufficient to synthesize significant amounts of vitamin D. If you have trouble getting outdoors much, or if it is often cloudy or rainy where you live, that's a problem, too. Also, if you have had problems with skin cancer and your dermatologist absolutely insists that you stay away from direct sunlight, then I strongly recommend

Latitude and Vitamin D

If you live at a latitude of 42 degrees (this would include Boston, Detroit, Chicago, central Iowa, and southern Oregon) you will probably make enough vitamin D from April to October to last throughout the year.

Below that, say in Washington, D.C., you have from March to November.

In the northern United States and Canada you have less time to make vitamin D, so you might want to consider taking a supplement.

that you make sure you get adequate vitamin D in your diet, or take a vitamin D supplement. I'll tell you more about how to get vitamin D into your diet and what kind of supplements to take, but first a word on vitamin D itself.

> **Sunshine and Vitamin D**
>
> Season, latitude, skin pigmentation, sunscreen, window glass, air pollution, and clothing can diminish the manufacture of vitamin D in the skin.

WHAT IS VITAMIN D?

Some people say that vitamin D is not really a vitamin at all, since it actually has the characteristics of a hormone. Vitamins, by definition, are organic substances that are essential for the proper growth and functioning of the body. They provide no calories, unlike carbohydrates, fat, and protein. They are absolutely necessary in small amounts for normal chemical reactions or metabolism inside the body. They must be obtained from food, because the body cannot manufacture them. That's funny, you might say, since I just told you that your body *can* make its own vitamin D when your skin is exposed to the UV rays in the sun. Right you are, and therein lies a slight classification problem.

Vitamins are essential to good health. When your vitamin intake is insufficient because of poor nutrition, restricted diet, or poor absorption in the intestine, then all kinds of diseases can occur. Some of the primary examples are:

O Anemia — due to vitamin B12 and folic acid deficiency

O Nerve and brain damage — due to vitamin B12 and thiamine deficiencies

O Excessive bleeding — due to vitamin K deficiency

O Blindness and poor night vision — due to vitamin A deficiency

O Scurvy — due to vitamin C deficiency

An addition to this list is bone disease, osteoporosis, and osteopenia, which results when our bodies are deficient in vitamin D and calcium (vitamin D being a vitamin or hormone, as we'll see, and calcium being a mineral, as we know). It is also interesting to note that alcoholics often develop a deficiency in niacin, thiamine, and folic acid. And sometimes, people on weight-loss drugs such as Xenical, which reduce the absorption of fat, develop deficiencies of the vitamins that normally dissolve in fat, namely vitamins A, D, E, and K.

Recently, researchers have come to believe that an inadequate intake of certain vitamins can cause diseases not usually attributed to vitamin deficiencies. For example, many doctors believe that an inadequate intake of vitamins B6, B12, and folic acid is associated with elevated levels of homocysteine, which can cause an increased risk of heart attack. We also now know that pregnant women who do not get adequate amounts of folic acid increase the risk of birth defects in their unborn children.

Vitamin D

Vitamin D can increase calcium absorption by up to 65%.

Doctors and patients have learned, to their dismay, that with some vitamins, too much of a good thing can be a bad thing. Vitamin A, for example, has recently been shown to be toxic in high levels, and to increase the risk of bone fracture by as much as 7% when taken in excess. A Swedish study published in the *New England Journal of Medicine* in January 2003 measured vitamin A (retinol) levels in blood samples from 2,300 men who were followed for up to thirty years, then compared the levels among the group. They found that men with the highest levels of vitamin A were 64% more likely to suffer a bone or hip fracture than those men with average levels of vitamin A. The risk of fracture was seven times higher among those with the highest levels of vitamin A, when compared with those with the lowest level.

A similar finding from the Nurses Health Study, which was an observational study of more than 72,000 nurses, showed that high intakes of vitamin A, specifically the retinol compound of this vitamin, may be associated with an increased risk of hip fracture. In fact, the hip fracture rate was double in the women who were taking more than 2,000 mcg of retinol (vitamin A) a day, when compared with the women taking only 500 mcg. These findings did not appear to apply to the beta-carotene form of vitamin A.

Vitamin A is made up of a group of substances that include retinol (a

preformed vitamin A) and carotenoids, substances that can be
converted into vitamin A. Retinol is used to form light-sensitive
nerve cells, or photoreceptors, in
the retina, and so helps us maintain normal vision. It also helps
maintain healthy skin, as well as
the health of the intestinal lining,
urinary tract, and lungs. It is the
basis for drugs called *retinoids,*
which are used to treat severe acne

> ## Vitamin A (Beta Carotene)
>
> Vitamin A (beta-carotene) can produce a small but significant increase in overall mortality and cardiovascular mortality, according to a 2003 study by doctors in Cleveland, published in *The Lancet.*

and even some cancers. The most plentiful form is retinol that is found
in animal foods, especially organs, meats, fish, fish oils, eggs, fortified cereals, and fortified milk. Carotenoids, which include beta-carotene, are found
in dark-green vegetables, and orange fruits and vegetables. Vitamin A supplements are made up of differing amounts of these forms of vitamin, so be
sure to check the label and remember that the beta-carotene form appears
to be safer.

Laura Tosi, M.D., a close friend of mine, is chair of the women's health
issues committee for the American Academy of Orthopaedic Surgeons. She
states that "we may have found a bone poison. Vitamin A is important in
small doses, but in high doses, it is poison."

More research is needed to find out just how much is too much vitamin
A, but the Swedish study suggests that consuming more than 1.5 mg per
day of retinol vitamin A from a supplement increases the risk of fracture.
The government is currently looking into how much vitamin A is safe as a
supplement in fortified cereals and multivitamin tablets, and manufacturers are beginning to reduce the amounts of vitamin A used in fortified foods
and multivitamins. Now for a brief look at hormones.

A hormone, by definition, is an active regulatory chemical substance
formed in one part of the body and carried by the bloodstream to another
part, where it signals the coordination of cellular functions. Among other
things, hormones are responsible for the development of secondary sexual
characteristics. Testosterone is the primary male hormone, and estrogen is the
primary female hormone. The biologically active form of vitamin D is a
hormone known as *calcitriol* (1,25DHCC), which I have already described.
It is sensitive to light and air, and is converted to vitamin D in the kidneys

Vitamin D Supplements

Vitamin D supplements *do not* need to be taken at the same time as calcium supplements. This is because the vitamin D stored in the body is converted to active forms, first by the liver and then the kidney, and can remain stable for days or even weeks.

Vitamin D Absorption

Mineral oil can destroy vitamin D in the intestines. Therefore, when used as a laxative, it interferes with calcium absorption.

before it can do its job. Because this fat-soluble vitamin is synthesized by the body itself, it is actually more like a hormone than a vitamin. Vitamin D3 is the natural form. It is called *cholecalciferol,* and is mostly found in fish oils. Vitamin D2 is the synthetic form, and it is known as *ergocalciferol.* When milk is fortified with vitamin D (a practice begun in the 1930s to help prevent rickets) either D3 or D2 can be used, but as I explained, it is the calcitriol that really does all the work when it comes to calcium absorption.

Whether you call it a vitamin or a hormone, vitamin D is essential for bone health, because it enables us to absorb calcium and phosphorus, thereby preserving the precious calcium-phosphorus balance in our blood. It also protects against bone loss by lowering excessive amounts of parathyroid hormone, which can increase to a dangerous level as we age. Vitamin D is fat soluble, so the body can store it for a long time. Recent studies have also indicated that adequate intakes of vitamin D may reduce the risk of breast cancer and colon cancer, and lower blood pressure by increasing calcium absorption. If you aren't able to get enough vitamin D in your diet, then you can make it yourself by exposing your skin to natural sunlight for five to fifteen minutes a day, when possible. You can also take supplements.

HOW MUCH VITAMIN D IS ENOUGH?

The amount of vitamin D you need depends on your age and where you live, but not on your gender. Young people living in sunny climates usually get all the vitamin D they need from the sun and the foods they eat. But research suggests that as we age, our ability to absorb vitamin D from our diet declines, just like our ability to absorb calcium. Also those with kidney or liver diseases need more vitamin D, since the liver and kidney are so important in turning inert vitamin D into active vitamin D. If you have liver or kidney problems, be sure to consult your physician on how to make sure you are getting all the vitamins and minerals you need.

> **The Kidney and Vitamin D**
>
> Levels of vitamin D in the kidney fall by about 40% as we age.

It also appears that after the age of sixty-five, our kidneys and liver no longer do such a good job of making active vitamin D. Because of this, the amount of calcium we absorb from our diet as we get older can decrease by as much as 40%.

Two studies conducted in the 1990s corroborate the evidence that vitamin D and calcium work well together as a team. In the first, researchers from Tufts University in 1991 found that giving patients 400 units of vitamin D3 along with 377 mg of calcium produces a slowdown of bone loss from the spine during the long winter months, when there was not enough sunlight for people to make the vitamin D they needed.

The second study, published in the *New England Journal of Medicine* in December 1992, described the findings of French researchers who had done a year-and-a-half-long study of women who were given 1,200 mg of calcium and 800 units of vitamin D3, compared with women who got neither calcium nor vitamin D.

> **The Liver and Vitamin D**
>
> Levels of vitamin D in our liver fall more than 50% as we age.

They found a 43% decrease in hip fracture in the group receiving the supplements.

As I said before, the amount of vitamin D you need depends on your age, and yet, menopause seems to have no effect on how much a woman needs. Therefore, the recommended amounts for women and men at a given age are the same. People over the age of seventy have the greatest need for vitamin D, and ironically they are less able to make it from sunlight. For many seniors it is not easy to get all the vitamin D they need from food, so I usually recommend a supplement. As you now know, there is strong evidence that adequate calcium and vitamin D intake in seniors may reduce the risk of bone fracture. As for how much each person needs, I usually recommend that my patients follow the guidelines established by the National Academy of Sciences in 1997:

Vitamin D Requirements for Men and Women

AGE	DAILY RECOMMENDED INTAKE
Birth to age 50	200 IU or 5 mcg
51 to 70	400 IU or 10 mcg
71 and older	600 IU or 15 mcg

(1 mcg = 40 IU or international units)

There is limited data available when it comes to measuring the exact amount of vitamin D in different foods. The vitamin D content differs depending on what kind of food the animal sources of vitamin D have been eating, what brand of food you buy, and just how much vitamin D has been added to fortified foods. Always read the label carefully for specific information.

The amount of vitamin D in a food product is not required on a label, so don't be surprised if you can't find a reference to the amount of vitamin D on a specific label.

How to Read a Food Label for Vitamin D Content

1. On a label, 100% Daily Value (%DV) is 400 IU per day.
2. Read the %DV for vitamin D per serving. For example, one serving of skim milk (8 ounces) contains 25% DV of vitamin D.
3. Calculate the vitamin D content (IU per serving). For example, 25% vitamin D = 25% of 400 IU = 100 IU per serving.

Food Sources of Vitamin D

Vitamin D occurs naturally in only a few foods:

- **Fatty fish,** including eel, salmon, bluefish, sardines and cod liver oil, herring, mackerel, shrimp, and oysters

- **Egg yolks**

- **Fortified foods,** including milk, soy milk, breakfast cereal, breakfast bars and rice milk (remember that most dairy products other than milk, yogurt, and cheese are usually not fortified with vitamin D)

- **Organ meats,** especially liver

- **Avocados**

- **Some mushrooms,** especially morels and shiitakes

Here's a breakdown of just how much vitamin D we can expect to get from certain amounts of those foods, as well as from vitamin D–fortified foods. Again, these quantities may vary, depending on the brand you buy or the diet of the particular fish or chicken you eat.

Sources of Vitamin D from Food	
	IU VITAMIN D PER SERVING
Herring, pickled	578 per 3 oz.
Salmon, pink, canned	530 per 3 oz.
Halibut	510 per 3 oz.
Catfish	425 per 3 oz.
Mackerel, Atlantic	306 per 3 oz.
Oyster	272 per 3 oz.
Shiitake mushrooms, dried	249 per 4 oz.
Sardines, Atlantic, in oil	203 per ½ cup
Tuna, light, in oil	200 per 3 oz.
Shrimp	129 per 3 oz.
Egg, cooked	26 per whole egg 25 per yolk

These days, we can also find a selection of foods fortified with vitamin D in the supermarket. Here is a list of some of these:

Foods Fortified with Vitamin D	
	IU VITAMIN D PER SERVING
Tofu, enriched	120 per ⅕ block
Cow's milk, all varieties	100 per 8 oz.
Milk, canned, evaporated	102 per 4 oz.
Soy milk, fortified	100 per 8 oz.
Pudding with fortified milk	50 per ½ cup
Cereal, fortified	40 per serving
Yogurt, fortified	40 per serving

When it comes to vitamin D supplements, there are three types. Multi-vitamins usually have 400 IU of vitamin D in them, but remember, they may be dangerously high in vitamin A, so be sure to read the label carefully to make sure you won't be getting too much vitamin A. Calcium with vitamin D supplements vary in the amount of vitamin D they contain, and so do the supplements containing only vitamin D. I purposely did not include cod liver oil, canned mackerel, and eel—as well as many other fish oils—in this list, because although they are high in vitamin D, they are also a major source of retinol vitamin A, which as I've pointed out before, appears to increase the risk of hip fracture in postmenopausal women, and in men, when taken in high doses.

WHAT DOES THIS HAVE TO DO WITH ME?

The bottom line on vitamin D is that it is essential for the absorption and use of calcium in our bodies. Vitamin D promotes the growth and maintenance of strong bones. We can get it in the foods we eat, in supplements, or easiest of all, by exposing our unprotected skin to sunlight for between five and fifteen minutes a day. From the ages of fifty-one to seventy, we need about 400 IU of vitamin D a day; after seventy we need about 600 to 800 IU a day. The irony—as with calcium—is that the older we get, the more we need, and the less able we are to manufacture it naturally from sunlight (or absorb it, in the case of calcium). Therefore, it is probably a good idea for everyone over fifty to take a supplement of either vitamin D alone, or a combination of calcium with vitamin D. And if you are over seventy, I'd say a vitamin D supplement is a must.

CHAPTER SEVEN

LITTLE THINGS
MEAN A LOT

*All About the Other "Must-Have" Nutrients
to Boost Calcium Absorption*

FOOD IS MADE UP **of six different elements:**

1. **Fluids,** which are essential to human life, **since 80% of the body is composed of water.**
2. **Carbohydrates,** which are our main source of energy. There are two types, complex and refined. **Complex carbohydrates** are the starches and fibers in foods such as vegetables, fruits, whole grains, nuts, legumes, seeds, and tubers. They are present in these foods just as they are found in nature, and they are good for us. They aid in digestion, help manufacture protein, and supply vitamins B and C. No one has fiddled with them. The second are **simple,** or **refined carbohydrates** such as sugar, which we get in cookies, cakes, candy, soft drinks, and other processed foods. These have been processed by machinery and are pale reflections of the carbohydrates found in nature. Refined carbohydrates have been stripped of their outer shell (the layer that contains most of the fiber), the oil, and the vitamin B–rich germ that is found in their core. They provide a huge percentage of our diet, yet they lack the essential vitamins, minerals, and fiber found in complex carbohydrates. They are bad for us, especially in the form of refined sugar, which can lead to obesity and diabetes. To say that they have been fiddled with a lot is putting it mildly.
3. **Protein,** which we need to repair human tissue. Sometimes proteins are high in fat and calories. Some of the food sources include meat, fish, milk, cheese, and nuts.

4. **Fats,** which help us absorb certain vitamins and give us energy. Unsaturated fats are healthier than saturated fats.
5. **Vitamins,** which are fundamental to health, growth, and sometimes disease prevention. We get them from plant and animal food sources, with the exception of vitamins D and K.
6. **Minerals,** which are chemicals required by the body to stay in good health. We do not manufacture these ourselves and must get them through food or supplements.

A batch of specific supplemental vitamins and minerals appears to be highly important for the absorption of calcium and for bone health in general.

The vitamins you need are:

○ Vitamin D (we've already discussed this in Chapter 6)

○ Vitamin C

○ Vitamin B
  • Vitamin B6
  • Vitamin B12
  • Folic acid (vitamin B9)

○ Vitamin K

The minerals you need are:

○ Boron

○ Calcium

○ Copper

○ Magnesium

○ Manganese

○ Phosphorus

○ Silica

○ Zinc

Don't get discouraged by the length of this list. Most of us get adequate amounts of these vitamins and minerals in our daily diet, and if we should show any signs of deficiency, all we need to do is take a supplement or improve our diet.

Before I describe each one of these—briefly, I promise—I'd like to explain just a little about vitamins and minerals in general. Vitamins are organic substances, which means that they contain carbon. I've always found it interesting that the only two pure forms of carbon on earth are diamonds, the hardest of all the gemstones, and graphite, that soft stuff used in the lead of your pencil. Vitamins are essential in small amounts for the normal growth and functioning of the cells in the body. They are obtained naturally from plant and animal foods. Although we need only small amounts of vitamins, they are absolutely essential to our health and well-being. In fact, without them, the higher animals, including us humans, could not exist. They affect all functions of the body and promote good vision, healthy bones and teeth, healthy blood cells, and proper functioning of the heart and central nervous system. They do not actually supply energy, but some of them do help with the efficient conversion of foods to energy.

There are thirteen vitamins essential to human health, and they fall into two categories:

VITAMINS

1. **Fat soluble: These are vitamins A, D, E, and K.** Just as the name implies, they are stored in your body's fat cells. All fat-soluble vitamins can be stored in the body for a long time, usually in the liver or fat tissue. Some of them, A and D in particular, can accumulate and reach toxic levels. This is why, as I mentioned in Chapter 6, you have to be careful when taking multivitamin pills.

2. **Water soluble: These include vitamin C and eight B vitamins**

   O **Vitamin B1 (thiamine)**

   O **Vitamin B2 (riboflavin)**

   O **Vitamin B3 (niacin)**

   O **Vitamin B5 (pantothenic acid)**

   O **Vitamin B6 (pyridoxine)**

   O **Vitamin B9 (folic acid)**

- **Vitamin B12 (cobalamin)**
- **Biotin**

The body does store these vitamins, but to a much lesser extent than the fat-soluble vitamins. Because of this, symptoms of deficiency in the water-soluble vitamins can show up quickly, within a few weeks to a month or so. The exception to this is B12, which can be stored for some time.

Vitamins are usually sensitive to heat and light, so keep them in a cool, dark place, or refrigerate them. Food will lose some of its vitamin content when it is being handled, stored, or cooked. Fat-soluble vitamins are more stable when being cooked than water-soluble ones. Boiling is particularly hard on water-soluble vitamins, so always boil vegetables in as little water as possible and for as short a time as possible. Better yet, steam them.

MINERALS

Your body needs minerals, too. Minerals are naturally occurring inorganic elements, meaning that they contain no carbon. They are the basic elements in the earth's crust. They are carried into the soil, groundwater, and sea by erosion, where plants absorb them and animals and humans ingest them by eating the plants. Actually, minerals account for about 4% of our body weight. The minerals in foods are not destroyed by cooking (heat), but boiling can leach out some of their minerals, so again it is smart to boil foods in as little water and for as short a time as possible. Also, minerals are often "processed" out of foods, as, for example, when whole grains are refined into flour.

Our bodies have more than sixty minerals, but only twenty-two of these are considered essential. Seven of these are called macrominerals, because they are in the body in large amounts. These are calcium, chloride, magnesium, phosphorus, potassium, sodium, and sulfur. The other essential minerals are called trace minerals because they occur in the body in such small amounts. The ones we need in larger amounts, and that are essential for our overall health, include:

- Calcium
- Phosphorus
- Magnesium

Those known as electrolytes, which regulate the water and chemical balance in the body, include:

O **Sodium**

O **Potassium**

O **Chloride**

Those minerals that play an essential role in bone health in particular are:

O **Boron**

O **Calcium**

O **Copper**

O **Magnesium**

O **Manganese**

O **Phosphorus**

O **Silica**

O **Zinc**

So much for the big picture. Now we'll take a quick look at those vitamins and minerals that you absolutely need for bone health, and why you need them. Remember:

1,000 micrograms (mcg) = 1 milligram
1,000 milligrams (mg) = 1 gram

Pay close attention to whether a recommended daily dosage is in **mg** or mcg. *There is a big difference.*

THE VITAMINS YOU NEED

Vitamin D

As explained in Chapter 6, we cannot absorb calcium without vitamin D, but we can get it from sunshine (which allows us to make it in our skin), through diet, or through supplements. We need about 400 to 800 IU of vitamin D a day, and it can be found in foods, including some fish liver oils, fatty fish, eggs (especially the yolks), vitamin D–fortified milk and bread, and chicken livers.

Vitamin C

We all know how important vitamin C is. Whole books have been written about the almost magical qualities of this water-soluble vitamin, which is able to boost the immune system, help heal wounds, and provide antioxidant properties that prevent cell damage by neutralizing "free radicals." Some studies even suggest that people who eat a lot of foods high in vitamin C lower their risk of cancer, heart disease, and age-related macular degeneration (AMD).

When it comes to bone health, vitamin C is essential for the formation of the cementlike substance that forms the internal supporting structure of the bone. Some observational studies have pointed to a possible relationship between vitamin C intake, bone mass, and reduced fracture risk, but so far no controlled clinical studies have done so. The Recommended Dietary Allowance is 125 mg a day for adult men and 90 mg a day for adult women. I think this is quite low.

Recommended dose: I usually recommend a minimum of 1,000 mg per day, which is quite easy to come by if you eat a healthy, well-balanced diet.

Toxic dose: 2,000 mg and above could cause diarrhea and intestinal upset.

Cautions: Do not take vitamin C if you have sickle-cell anemia, kidney stones, gout, or iron-deficiency disease.

Food Sources for Vitamin C	
Citrus fruits: oranges, grapefruit, lemons, limes	Cabbage
	Raw peppers
Tomatoes	Broccoli
Cantaloupe	Potatoes

The B Vitamins

B6, B12, and folic acid (B9)

Vitamin B6 (Pyridoxine)

This water-soluble vitamin plays an important but indirect role in the metabolism of bone. B6 is necessary for the production of hydrochloric acid (HCl), and HCl helps with calcium absorption. B6 has been shown to work together with B12 and folic acid to reduce the levels of homocysteine in the blood.

When homocysteine levels get too high, the risk of heart attack, stroke, or loss of circulation in your hands and feet go up. B6 is also essential for the proper function of the adrenal glands, which produce some thirty hormones that, among other things, help maintain proper mineral balance in the body. Animal studies have shown that animals with vitamin B6 deficiency form less, and lower quality, new bone than those with adequate levels of the vitamin. A British study found B6 deficiency more common among people who suffer hip fractures than among those who don't.

Recommended dose: The RDA for adults over fifty is 1.7 mg per day for men and 1.5 mg per day for women.

Toxic dose: A maximum intake of 100 mg per day from all sources is unlikely to pose risks for adults.

Cautions: Consult with your doctor before taking vitamin B6 if you have intestinal problems, liver disease, sickle-cell disease, an overactive thyroid, or if you have been under a lot of stress because of surgery, an accident, illness, or burns.

Food Sources for Vitamin B6	
Wheat and corn products	Beef
Yeast	Pork
Soybeans	Poultry
Lima beans	Organ meats

Vitamin B12 (Cobalamin)

B12, another water-soluble vitamin, is on the list of essential nutrients for good bone health. Without adequate B12, our osteoblasts can't do their job. B12 is not found in plant foods, and sometimes, vegetarians can develop a deficiency in this vitamin. It plays an essential role in red blood cell formation, cell metabolism, and nerve function. It is estimated that 10 to 30% of adults over fifty have a B12 deficiency because they can't absorb food-bound vitamin B12. Large amounts of B12 are stored in the liver, so it can take years for a deficiency to show up. People who have pernicious anemia or who have had gastrointestinal surgery may require injections of B12.

Recommended dose: The RDA for adult men and women is 2.4 mcg per day.

Toxic dose: There is no known toxicity in humans from vitamin B12.

Cautions: Check with your doctor before taking B12 if you have anemia from no known cause.

Food Sources for Vitamin B12

Meat	Beans
Fish	Lentils
Shellfish	Tofu
Poultry	Nuts
Eggs	Organ meats
Dairy products	Some fortified cereals
Cheese	

Vitamin B9 (Folic Acid/Folate)

Folic acid is the synthetic form of folate. Folic acid is found in fortified cereals, fortified breads, and supplements. It is another water-soluble vitamin, and it is important in red blood cell formation, protein metabolism, growth, and cell division. It is extremely important to the developing fetus in pregnant women.

Recommended dose: The RDA for both men and women is 400 mcg per day. For pregnant women it is 600 mcg per day.

Toxic dose: Intake from fortified foods should not be over 1,000 mcg a day, in order to prevent folic acid from covering up a vitamin B12 deficiency.

Cautions: Check with your doctor if you have anemia. Folic acid may cause bright yellow urine, fever, shortness of breath, a skin rash, and, rarely, diarrhea. Doses over 1,500 mcg per day can cause appetite loss, nausea, flatulence, and a distended abdomen.

Food Sources of Folic Acid (Folate)	
Citrus juices	Cereals, fortified
Fruits	Rice, fortified
Nuts	Beans
Seeds	Liver
Beans	Dark-green, leafy vegetables
Pasta, fortified	

Vitamin K

In addition to its important role in blood clotting, vitamin K is also necessary for the body to make a protein, osteocalcin, that plays an important role in binding calcium crystals in the bone. Osteocalcin gives structure and order to your bone tissue, thereby giving bone its strength. The protein also helps bind calcium to the bone matrix. One study found that circulating vitamin K was lower in patients who had had osteoporatic bone fractures than in those who had no fractures. In a Japanese study, vitamin K was given to postmenopausal women over a period of two years, and it reduced their calcium loss to 18% from as high as 50%. A study in the Netherlands confirmed this study. In this study, 25% of the healthy postmenopausal women evaluated had elevated excretion of calcium in their urine, suggesting that they were losing bone quickly. When they took vitamin K, the unwanted calcium loss was reduced by one third, suggesting that the bone loss was also reduced by one third. Before the women in the second study started to take vitamin K, the capacity of their osteocalcin to attract calcium was reduced. After taking 1 mg of vitamin K every day for two weeks, this bone protein started working normally again.

In the U.S. Nurses' Health Study, in which the diet of 72,327 women was analyzed, it showed that those women eating one or more servings of lettuce (a good source of vitamin K) every day reduced the risk of hip fracture by 45%.

Vitamin K also appears to play a major role in the healing of fractures. In one study, the bone fractures of rabbits given a vitamin K supplement healed more quickly than those in rabbits not given the vitamin K. When humans break a bone, their vitamin K levels fall during recovery, suggesting that the K is being drawn from the rest of the blood to the site of the fracture.

Vitamin K (like vitamin D) is produced in the body. Vitamin K is produced by certain healthy intestinal bacteria.

Recommended dose: The RDA has been set for between 90 and 120 mcg per day for adults. I recommend between 100 and 300 mcg per day.

Cautions: Excessive amounts of man-made vitamin K can cause jaundice, a yellowing of the skin. Antibiotics can destroy the intestinal bacteria that produce vitamin K. The ability of vitamin K to be effective is threatened by mineral oil laxatives, the freezing of food, radiation, impaired fat absorption, sulfa drugs, and certain liver diseases.

Food Sources of Vitamin K

Liver	Green tea
Green, leafy vegetables	Asparagus
Cabbage	Green peas
Milk	Green beans
Eggs	Whole wheat
Cereals	Oats
Meat	

THE MINERALS YOU NEED

Boron

Boron has been getting more and more attention lately. We used to think that boron was only useful as a food preservative in the form of boric acid. By the 1950s it became clear that people consuming more than 500 mg of boron per day developed appetite and general health problems, and it was outlawed worldwide as a food preservative. Recently, however, the story has dramatically changed. We now know that the body requires boron to metabolize and use various bone-building agents, including calcium, magnesium, vitamin D, estrogen, and maybe even testosterone. Here are some impressive results of recent studies:

○ In 1987, Dr. Forest Neilsen of the U.S. Department of Agriculture Research Service in Grand Forks, North Dakota, conducted a study that found that when postmenopausal women took a boron supplement, their metabolism of calcium and magnesium improved. Those studied lost 44% less calcium from their bodies, 33% less magnesium, and slightly less phosphorus after taking 3 mg of boron for seven weeks than the women who didn't take the supplement. What's more, after taking boron supplements for eight days, the blood levels of bone-building estrogen and testosterone nearly doubled. The effects of boron were most pronounced in women with low magnesium levels. His follow-up study in 1995 did not duplicate these findings, but research continues, and many nutritionists feel that boron plays an important role in bone health.

○ Later studies have found that boron supplements raise 17 beta-estradiol levels of women on estrogen therapy. Although the results of his original study have not been repeated, Dr. Neilsen does feel that women on hormone therapy might get along with a lower dose if they take boron supplements. Dr. Neilsen subsequently gave postmenopausal women boron to see if it could reduce the symptoms of menopause, including hot flashes. These women took 3 mg of boron per day. In 25% of the women hot flashes improved; in 50% there were no noticeable changes; in 25% hot flashes got worse. It is clear that more research needs to be done to find out just what the boron-estrogen connection is, and how it works.

Recommended dose: No RDA has been established, but recent research suggests that 2 to 3 mg per day is probably the optimum intake.

Toxic dose: More than 3 mg from supplements could be dangerous and have a negative effect on calcium metabolism. There is no restriction on boron from foods—in fact, people in some parts of the world get as much as 41 mg in their diet every day.

Food Sources of Boron

Vegetables	Applesauce (canned)
Avocado	Cherries
Broccoli	Grape juice
Carrots	Grapes
Celery	Oranges
Parsley (dried)	Peaches
Squash	Pears
Spinach (canned)	Plums
Legumes (cooked)	Prune juice
Black-eyed peas	Prunes
Lima beans	Raisins (dried)
Pinto beans	Strawberries
Kidney beans	Nuts and seeds
Fruits	Almonds
Apples (red)	Peanuts, peanut butter
Apple juice (canned)	Wine

Calcium

Everything you have ever wanted to know about this bone-building essential, calcium, can be found in Chapter 5.

Copper

Copper is an essential trace mineral. Only recently has it been found to be important in maintaining bone health. This was discovered when professional basketball star Bill Walton kept breaking bones even though he was a young, healthy athlete. When doctors analyzed his diet they found it lacking in the trace minerals zinc,

Copper Deficiency

The average American diet contains only 50% of the RDA for copper. One study found that all segments of the population have a copper deficiency ranging from 50 to 83% of the RDA.

copper, and manganese. When he started taking supplements of these minerals, along with calcium, his condition was cured. Although we are not sure exactly how copper works in bone health, we do know that it is an aid in the formation of collagen for bone and connective tissue. Inadequate levels of copper, as well as manganese, have been associated with osteoporosis.

Recommended dose: 1.5 to 3 mg per day for everyone over eleven.

Cautions: Copper excretion will be increased by a diet high in sugar and refined flour. There is some evidence that lactose, the sugar in milk, interferes with copper metabolism. A diet high in dairy products could decrease the utilization of copper.

Food Sources of Copper		
Filberts	Liver	Oysters
Pecans	Lamb	Seafood
Peanuts	Pork	Cereals
Walnuts	Legumes	

Magnesium

This mineral (a trace element) is important in many enzyme processes. It is a component of all cells and helps with bone formation, protein synthesis, muscle function, and regulation of body temperature and blood pressure. There are approximately 25 grams of magnesium in our body, and half is in our bones. A study in 1998 found that the symptoms of premenstrual syndrome were reduced by 40% in women who took 200 mg of magnesium per day. Infusions of magnesium have also been successful in the treatment of pain associated with migraine headaches in some patients.

Although magnesium deficiency is rare, certain diuretics can cause excessive amounts of it to be excreted in the urine. Thiazide diuretics, often used to treat high blood pressure, heart failure, and fluid retention, are culprits in magnesium loss. It is often difficult to know when someone is magnesium deficient, because blood levels of this mineral do not accurately reflect how much magnesium is stored in the body until that depletion is severe. Doctors may prescribe a magnesium supplement for patients on thiazide drugs.

Magnesium has a role in the production of a bone hormone called parathyroid hormone (PTH). When magnesium is low, less PTH is released. Normal levels of PTH cause bone to be produced, but high levels of PTH cause calcium to be leached from bone. Scientists agree that more research is necessary to pin down the exact role of magnesium when it comes to bone health.

Food Sources of Magnesium

Green, leafy vegetables
Legumes (dried beans)
Whole grains
Nuts and seeds
Seafood
Milk
Yogurt

Recommended dose: Women thirty-one and older, 320 mg per day; men thirty-one and older, 420 mg per day. When taken with food, unpleasant side effects such as nausea, diarrhea, and stomach cramps are less likely to occur. The risk of unpleasant side effects tends to go up after the age of fifty-five.

Toxic dose: Too much magnesium can cause diarrhea. Notice what happens when you take Milk of Magnesia.

Cautions: Do not take magnesium if you are pregnant, breast-feeding, have kidney failure or heart block (unless you have a pacemaker). Check with your doctor about magnesium if you have colitis, diarrhea, chronic constipation, stomach or intestinal bleeding, or symptoms of appendicitis.

Manganese

Manganese is another trace element. We need it in very small amounts for proper nutrition. The trick with all trace elements is that toxic levels can be only two or three times the recommended daily intake, so you usually need a doctor's supervision before taking them as a supplement. Manganese was one of the trace elements that Bill Walton was deficient in when he started having osteoporosis-related bone fractures. It turns out that this deficiency was due to the fact that he had been on an unusual, highly restricted diet.

It appears that manganese deficiency is critical to the development of cartilage and bone. Most of the research on this element has been done in animals, not humans, but people with osteoporosis do sometimes have a manganese deficiency. New research has shown that manganese deficiency seems to increase bone breakdown, while at the same time it decreases new bone mineralization. Meanwhile, decreased bone breakdown has been shown

Food Sources of Manganese

Liver
Kidney
Red meats
Spinach
Lettuce
Legumes (dried beans
    and peas)
Nuts
Whole grains

to correlate with higher blood serum levels of manganese. One study in particular showed that women with osteoporosis had only one quarter of the manganese levels of women who did not have osteoporosis.

Here's an interesting little fact. Manganese has replaced lead in gasoline. This means that there is more manganese in the air as a kind of pollutant. There should, as a result of this, be more manganese in foods now, so that a deficiency is less likely now than ever. Too much manganese can cause a generalized disease of the central nervous system, so it is probably not wise to take it as a supplement unless specifically recommended by your doctor.

Recommended dose: No RDA has been established, but the official recommendation for a "safe and adequate" amount of manganese is between 3.5 and 7 mg for adults.

Cautions: An excessively high intake of manganese can cause a generalized disease of the central nervous system.

Phosphorus

Phosporus is the second most abundant mineral in the body. It plays a big role in all chemical reactions, including cell growth and repair, energy production, nerve and muscle activity, heart contraction, and in the metabolism of calcium, glucose, starch, and fat. What is important about phosphorus in the bone department is that it combines with calcium to form a mineral salt that gives structure and strength to our bones and teeth. In fact, 80% of our total body phosphorus is located in our bones and teeth. Although phosphorus is imperative to good bone health, as well as to our health in general, too much of it can be bad. It is all about balance. The optimum ratio of calcium to phosphorus is 1:1. What happens is that we get so much phosphorus in our diet, especially from soft drinks and processed foods, that the balance gets out of whack and the ratio can go up to 2:1, 3:1, or even 4:1 when measured against our calcium intake. This high phosphorus-to-calcium ratio can cause serious damage to our bones, so it is most important to try to keep the ratio within the 1:1 range.

Recommended Dose: The current RDA suggests that the ratio between calcium and phosphorus be close to 1:1, so if you are getting 1,200 mg of calcium per day, you can also allow yourself 1,200 mg of phosphorus. Be careful, though. It is easy for the phosphorus number (in the form of phosphoric acid) to soar, because there is so much of it in the soft drinks and processed foods we Americans tend to eat in such great quantities.

Cautions: As long as your kidneys are healthy, and you keep your calcium-to-phosphorus ratio close to 1:1, there shouldn't be a problem with toxicity. Because phosphorus is found in nearly all the foods we eat, and is especially high in meat and soft drinks, most people get more than they need in their diet, and taking it in supplement form is not necessary.

> **Food Sources of Phosphorus**
>
> Meat
> Meat products
> Soft drinks
> Dairy products
> Processed foods (especially baked goods)
> Cheese to which phosphorus compounds have been added

> **Processed Foods**
>
> A shocking 80% of the foods Americans eat today are processed foods. In 1900, only 10% of the foods we ate were processed. Any food with a label on it is probably a processed food.

Silica

Silica is the most abundant mineral on earth. We don't know a whole lot about how it actually works in the body, but we do know that it is abundant in our stronger tissues such as nails, hair, teeth, tendons, arteries, skin, connective tissue, and collagen. Bone collagen increases with silica supplementation, and silica also strengthens our connective tissue matrix by cross-linking our strands of collagen. When our calcium levels are low, silica appears to increase bone mineralization. Silica then seems to initiate the calcification process in the bone, thereby keeping our bones strong and flexible. As I said, more research is still needed to figure out just how all this works, but the relationship between healthy bones and silica is clear.

Recommended dose: There is no established RDA for silica, but research suggests that adults need from 20 to 30 mg per day.

Cautions: When you eat a lot of processed food, you lower your body's intake of silica. Try to keep your diet full of fresh fruits, vegetables, and whole grains.

Food sources of Silica	
Mother's milk	Parsnips
Brown rice	Cucumbers
Barley	Onions
Oats	Whole grains
Green, leafy vegetables	Fruits (especially the skins)
Bell peppers	Nuts and seeds
Leeks	Beans

Zinc

Zinc is a heavy hitter when it comes to bone health. Here are some of the things it does:

O It acts as a "cofactor" in more than two hundred enzyme reactions.

O It is part of the matrix of collagen protein threads that puts the bone-forming calcium-phosphorus compound on the bone.

O It is necessary for calcium absorption.

O It enhances the chemical activity of vitamin D.

O It is essential for bone healing.

Low levels of zinc have been associated with osteoporosis. In one study, women with osteoporosis had 30% less zinc in their bloodstream than nonosteoporatic women. The bone-zinc levels in these same women were 28% lower than in the healthy women. People with advanced jawbone loss also have lower levels of zinc in their bloodstream.

Recommended dose: The current RDA level for adult men is 15 mg per day; for adult women it is 12 mg per day.

Cautions: Most Americans are probably zinc deficient. One estimate is that only 8% of us are getting the amount of zinc we need. Another study, conducted by the Massachusetts Institute of Technology, estimated that 68% of us consume less than two thirds of the zinc we need each day. Women and teenage girls have the lowest zinc consumption of all.

Food Sources of Zinc	
Whole grains, bran, wheat, wheat germ	Nuts, cashews, peanuts, pecans, pumpkin seeds, sesame seeds, sunflower seeds
Zinc-fortified cereals	
Bran flakes, oatmeal, raisin bran, raisin rice, and rye	Beef
	Chicken
	Eggs
Legumes (dried beans and peas)	Lamb
	Lobster
Milk	Oysters
Cheese	Pork

THIS MAY BE MORE than you ever wanted to know about vitamins and minerals, but since they are so important to bone health, let me try to simplify all this information. Nutritionists almost always agree that the best source of vitamins and minerals is the foods we eat. They don't always agree on how much you should take of these vitamins and minerals in the form of supplements. This, of course, depends on how healthy you are and how varied your overall diet is, and I would always advise you to check with your doctor before starting on any supplements. In general, though, I feel that the following supplement breakdown works well for most of my patients:

Dr. Root's Essential Vitamin Recommendations

VITAMIN	DAILY DOSAGE
Vitamin A (as beta-carotene)	3,000 mcg (equals 10,000 IU)
B Vitamins	
Vitamin B6	1.7 mg, men 1.5 mg, women
Vitamin B12	2.4 mcg, men and women
Vitamin B9 (Folic Acid)	400 mcg, men and women
Vitamin C	1,000 mg, divided, men and women
Vitamin D	400–800 IU, men and women
Vitamin E	400 IU, men and women
Vitamin K	100–300 mcg, men and women

Dr. Root's Essential Mineral Recommendations

MINERAL	DAILY DOSAGE
Boron	2–3 mcg, men and women
Calcium	1,200-1,500 mg, men and women
Copper	2.5–10 mg, men and women
Magnesium	600–750 mg (2:1 ratio with calcium)
Manganese	3.5–7 mg, men and women
Phosphorus	800–1,500 mg (1:1 ratio with calcium; not taken as a supplement)
Silica	20–30 mg, men and women
Zinc	12 mg, women 15 mg, men

Some nutritionists and medical professionals who deal with osteoporosis recommend dosages as high as 5,000 to 10,000 IU of vitamin A, 4 mg of boron, 800 mg of magnesium, 25 mg of manganese, 1,000 mg of silica, and 25 mg of zinc. I believe that my more conservative numbers are safer and perfectly adequate.

A Word About Supplements

Every five years the U.S. government publishes an updated list of the amount of various food elements they believe should be included in a healthy average American diet. They call this *Nutrition and Your Health: Dietary Guidelines for Americans,* and a new one is scheduled for release in 2005. You can learn more about this on the web at http://www.health.gov/dietaryguidelines/. Based on these guidelines, many foods are required to have their nutritional value shown on the label. The Food and Drug Administration (FDA) lists these requirements on their website at http://www.cfsan.fda.gov/~dms/lab-cons.html. In order to better understand these labeling requirements, you should understand a few terms:

- **DRI (Dietary Reference Intake):** This is the new term for the U.S. RDA, recommended dietary allowance, of essential vitamins, minerals, and, in some cases, protein. It is the general term for the guidelines that now cover all of the items that follow. DRIs have been established for seventeen vitamins and minerals, as well as for beta-carotene and other carotenoids, specifically those that enter the body and are converted into vitamin A.

- **RDA (Recommended Dietary Allowance):** This represents the estimated nutrient allowance necessary for a healthy person, established by the National Academy of Sciences and updated periodically to reflect the most recent findings in the field of nutrition. Sometimes RDAs differ for men, women, and according to age group. The term has now been replaced by DRI.

- **AI (Adequate Intake):** When researchers decide that there is not enough data to establish an RDA, they settle for an AI, which is a rougher estimate than an RDA.

- **UL (Tolerable Upper Intake Level):** The highest level one can safely take without unpleasant or dangerous side effects.

- **EAR (Estimated Average Requirement):** This refers to the amount of a nutrient that meets the requirement of half of a particular group, such as women over fifty, for example. This number is used to help calculate the RDA/DRI.

O **DV (Daily Value):** This is a new term that will appear on food labels. It is made up of two sets of references, DRV and DRI.

O **DRV (Daily Reference Value):** This is the dietary reference that tells you how much fat, saturated fat, cholesterol, carbohydrate, sodium, fiber, and potassium is in a given food.

WHAT DOES THIS HAVE TO DO WITH ME?

Are you confused enough yet? Don't worry. Just look at the label on the packaged foods and supplements you buy. If it says RDA, simply remember that these estimates are on the low side of what experts now think are more acceptable levels of the nutrients we need every day. If it says DRI, you're in business. Those estimates represent a more up-to-date assessment of the adequate amount of various vitamins and minerals needed in a balanced diet.

The Office of Dietary Supplements (ODS), a part of the National Institutes of Health, is the official U.S. agency dedicated to finding "new knowledge to help prevent, detect, diagnose and treat disease and disability, from the rarest genetic disorder to the common cold." They point out that in Asia and Europe, many studies of dietary supplements are being conducted, especially on supplements derived from "natural" or plant sources. But they say that the majority of these supplements have not been scientifically studied. You can learn more about what the ODS is doing in the area of supplement research at their website, which you can find through http://www.nih.gov/.

Meanwhile, before you purchase any dietary supplement, be sure to read the label carefully. This applies to the foods you buy, as well, because as I said at the beginning of this chapter, the best source of all the nutrients we need is in the foods we eat. Sometimes, though, vitamin and mineral supplements can be your insurance policy. If you have any reason to believe that your diet may be insufficient in any important nutrient, then try to get it in a supplement, according to the guidelines I've suggested in this chapter.

CHAPTER EIGHT

THE GOOD,
THE NOT SO GOOD,
AND THE TERRIBLE

Which Foods to Eat; Which to Cut Down On;
Which to Avoid Like the Plague

WHICH FOODS TO EAT

LET'S KEEP IT SIMPLE. Here is a list of foods that are healthy, nutritious, high in calcium, and great additions to your diet. Just a little reminder, though: We are only able to absorb a small amount of the calcium we take in. When I recommend that all adults over fifty try to get 1,500 mg of calcium into their diets each day, I realize that you will not be able to absorb all that calcium. The recommended daily allowances issued by the government and other nutritional institutions take this into account, too. How much calcium you actually absorb depends on your age, your digestive system, what other foods you are eating (or not eating), and what medications you might be taking. For now, just try to follow the general guidelines, eat (or take in supplement form) at least 1,500 mg of calcium per day, and you will be doing your body and your bones a great favor.

How do you do that? We'll start out with dairy products, the foods with the highest calcium content of all. These foods can also be high in fat, so try to use a low-fat variety whenever possible.

Low-fat dairy products actually contain more calcium than those that still have their fat. What happens is that the calcium in dairy products becomes more concentrated when the fat has been taken out. Some of the volume previously taken up by fat is now replaced by other nutrients, in-

For the Lactose-Intolerant

You can buy milk with lactase enzymes added. These break down the lactose that causes the problem. You can also buy enzymes separately and add them to or take them along with dairy products.

Calcium in the Average American Diet

Most Americans eat only between 250 and 600 mg of calcium a day. These people tend to be deficient in other important vitamins and minerals, too. Increasing calcium-rich foods can increase other important nutrients, as well, including those essential to healthy, beautiful bones.

cluding calcium. When you have a low-fat dairy product, it will be higher in essential nutrients, including calcium, than its whole-milk counterpart.

Most of us know that it is important to keep our diet fairly low in fat to protect our heart and reduce the risk of stroke, cancer, and obesity. Until the age of about two, children need fat, so they should drink whole milk, but for those of us over two, nonfat dairy products are a good idea. Skim milk has more calcium than whole milk, as I have explained. It is also interesting that plain, nonfat yogurt has even more calcium than milk, but yogurt has no added vitamin D, so keep that in mind when deciding which of the high-calcium dairy products to include in your diet. I believe that it is a good idea to have milk on your cereal in the morning and yogurt as a snack sometime during the day, and to add grated hard cheese to your vegetables or salad at dinner. This can help you jump-start your calcium intake every day. I'll discuss this in more detail in Chapters 9 and 10. Now, here is a list of some of the best high-calcium, low-fat dairy products going. I've included some whole dairy products, too, so you can compare them with the low-fat group. The following measurements are approximate, and are based on a study published in November 1999 by the U.S. Department of Agriculture, called *Nutrient Database for Standard Reference.*

DAIRY PRODUCT	AMOUNT OF CALCIUM
MILK (mg of calcium in 1 cup milk)	
Whole milk (5% milk-fat)	291 mg
Low-fat 2% (with vitamins A and D added)	297 mg
Low-fat 1% (with vitamins A and D added)	300 mg
Nonfat (with vitamins A and D added)	302 mg
Whole dry milk	1,168 mg
Nonfat dry milk	1,508 mg
Condensed, sweetened	868 mg
Evaporated milk	658 mg
Evaporated nonfat milk	738 mg
Chocolate milk	280 mg
Eggnog	330 mg
Goat's milk	326 mg
CREAM (mg of calcium in 1 cup cream)	
Whipping cream, heavy	154 mg
Whipping cream, light	166 mg
Whipping cream, pressurized	61 mg
Half and half	254 mg
Sour cream	268 mg
Ice cream, vanilla	170 mg
Sherbet, orange	80 mg
YOGURT (mg of calcium in 1 cup yogurt)	
Plain, whole milk	274 mg
Plain, low-fat	415 mg
Plain, nonfat	452 mg
Fruit, low-fat	314 mg
CHEESE (mg of calcium in 1 ounce cheese)	
Blue cheese	150 mg
Brie	52 mg
Camembert	110 mg
Cheddar	204 mg
Cheshire	182 mg
Cottage cheese, creamed (1 cup)	135 mg
Cottage cheese, low-fat (1%; 1 cup)	137 mg
Cream cheese	23 mg
Edam	207 mg

Feta	140 mg
Fontina	156 mg
Gouda	198 mg
Gruyère	287 mg
Limburger	141 mg
Monterey Jack	212 mg
Mozzarella	147 mg
Mozzarella (part skim)	183 mg
Muenster	203 mg
Parmesan (hard)	336 mg
Parmesan (grated)	138 mg
Port du Salut	184 mg
Provolone	214 mg
Ricotta (1 cup)	509 mg
Ricotta (1 cup, part skim)	669 mg
Romano	302 mg
Roquefort	188 mg
Swiss	272 mg
Swiss, processed	219 mg
American, processed	174 mg
American cheese spread	159 mg

Twenty-four-Hour Calcium

Consider eating a calcium-rich snack like yogurt at bedtime to provide calcium at night, since your body needs calcium twenty-four hours a day.

Low-Calcium Cheeses

Cream cheese and cottage cheese (unless you get an enriched brand) are not particularly good sources of calcium.

It is certainly clear that dairy products, especially yogurt, ricotta, and parmesan cheese are great sources of calcium. If you are lactose-intolerant, try purchasing brands that have enzymes added, buy helpful enzymes separately and add them, or take them at the same time you eat your low-fat dairy foods. A whole egg, by the way, contains 28 mg of calcium, twenty-six of which are in the yolk. Eggs are also loaded with other important nutrients, including magnesium and vitamin D.

Fruits

Although fruits are not particularly high in calcium (with a few exceptions), I'm going to list some of them here because they are so important to our health. I have long been convinced that the healthiest overall diet by far is one containing lots of fresh fruits, fresh vegetables, and low-fat dairy products. By eating in this way, you can usually get all the vitamins, minerals, and nutrients you need, naturally, from the foods themselves. One of the reasons natural foods are superior to supplements is that one food is often able to provide dozens of essential vitamins, minerals, and nutrients all by itself. Just look at an avocado, for example. One medium-sized avocado gives you 1,204 mg of potassium, 1,230 IU of vitamin A, 79 mg of magnesium, 22 mg of calcium, as well as healthy quantities of many other essential vitamins and minerals. That's not bad for one little fruit. It is, of course, important to keep fats and carbohydrates and even protein to a minimum if you want to maximize your calcium absorption, but you already knew that.

> **Dried Figs**
>
> One cup of dried figs contains a whopping 269 mg of calcium. Try chopping them up and adding them to cereal or salads.

FRUIT AND FRUIT JUICE	CALCIUM
(mg of calcium in 1 cup unless otherwise specified)	
Apple (1 medium)	10 mg
Apple juice	16 mg
Applesauce, unsweetened	7 mg
Apricot (3)	15 mg
Apricot nectar	17 mg
Avocado (1)	22 mg
Banana (1 medium)	7 mg
Blackberries	46 mg
Blueberries	9 mg
Boysenberries (frozen)	36 mg
Cherries (without pits)	21 mg
Cherries (sour)	16.5 mg
Cranberries	7 mg
Currants, black	61 mg

Dates (10)	**27 mg**
Elderberries	**55 mg**
Figs	**22 mg**
Figs, dried	**269 mg**
Grapefruit (½ medium)	**14 mg**
Grapefruit juice	**22 mg**
Grapes, seedless	**17 mg**
Grape juice	**22 mg**
Kiwi (1 medium)	**20 mg**
Kumquat (1)	**8 mg**
Lemon juice (1 tablespoon)	**2 mg**
Lime juice (1 tablespoon)	**1 mg**
Loganberries, frozen	**38 mg**
Mango (1)	**21 mg**
Melon (cantaloupe, small)	**49 mg**
Melon (honeydew, ¼ slice)	**20 mg**
Mulberries	**55 mg**
Nectarine (1)	**6 mg**
Orange (1)	**52 mg**
Orange juice	**27 mg**
Papaya (1)	**72 mg**
Peach	**5 mg**
Peach, dried (10 halves)	**37 mg**
Peach nectar	**13 mg**
Pear (1)	**19 mg**
Pear, dried (10 halves)	**59 mg**
Pear nectar	**11 mg**
Persimmon (1)	**13 mg**
Pineapple	**11 mg**
Pineapple juice	**42 mg**
Plantain	**4 mg**
Plum	**2 mg**
Pomegranate	**5 mg**
Prune (10)	**43 mg**
Prune juice	**30 mg**
Quince (1)	**10 mg**
Raisin, packed	**46 mg**
Raspberries	**27 mg**

Rhubarb	**105 mg**
Strawberries	**21 mg**
Tangerine (1 mandarin)	**12 mg**
Tangerine juice	**44 mg**
Watermelon	**13 mg**

If you really want to load up on calcium through fresh fruits or fruit juices, try tangerine juice (44 mg), rhubarb (105 mg), ten prunes (43 mg), pineapple juice (42 mg), a papaya (72 mg), an orange (52 mg), a small cantaloupe (49 mg), black currants (61 mg), blackberries (46 mg), or really go for it with dried figs, at an impressive 269 mg of calcium per cup.

Fruits: Good, and Good for You

Fruits are sweet (containing combined sugars of fructose, glucose, and sucrose) and low in calories, because most fruits are 80 to 95% water. They provide fiber (apples, pears, dates, and figs), and except for avocados and bananas, are almost fat-free and cholesterol-free. They also provide vitamin C, and yellow and orange fruits, such as apricots, cantaloupes, peaches, nectarines, and mangoes, are great sources of beta-carotene, the precursor of vitamin A.

Citrus Juice

Citrus juices are high in vitamin C, which deteriorates when in contact with oxygen. To prevent this, store them in tightly closed glass containers. Also make sure the label says 100% juice. Otherwise, you might be getting lots of water and sugar and very little juice.

"Fruit-Vegetables"

Although we refer to them as vegetables, eggplants, squash, peppers, and tomatoes are actually fruits, because the fleshy part of the plant contains seeds. They are high in vitamin C, and are used as seasonings and accents (tomato paste, chili sauce, catsup), as well as staple foods.

Cancer-Fighting Vegetables

Cruciferous vegetables—including cabbage, broccoli, brussels sprouts, kale, cauliflower, collard greens, mustard greens, rutabagas, and turnips—contain nitrogen compounds called indoles, which appear effective in fighting cancer, especially of the stomach and large intestine.

Calcium Interactions

The calcium in spinach and rhubarb is almost completely unavailable because they are so high in oxalates. Beet greens and almonds are high in oxalates too.

VEGETABLES AND VEGETABLE JUICES	CALCIUM
(mg of calcium in 1 cup unless otherwise stated)	
Artichoke (1 globe)	61 mg
Artichoke (1 Jerusalem)	21 mg
Arugula	32 mg
Asparagus	28 mg
Beet greens	46 mg
Beets	22 mg
Broccoli	42 mg
Brussels sprouts	36 mg
Cabbage, common	32 mg
Cabbage, Chinese	74 mg
Carrot juice	8.3 mg
Carrots	30 mg
Cauliflower	28 mg
Celery	44 mg
Chard, Swiss	18 mg
Chicory greens	180 mg
Collard greens	52 mg
Corn	4 mg
Cucumber	14 mg
Dandelion greens	103 mg

Eggplant	30 mg
Endive	26 mg
Garlic (1 clove)	5 mg
Green beans	41 mg
Kale	90 mg
Kohlrabi	34 mg
Leeks	73 mg
Lettuce, iceberg	15 mg
Lettuce, romaine	20 mg
Mushrooms	4 mg
Mushrooms, portobello	8 mg
Mustard greens	58 mg
Okra	82 mg
Onion greens	60 mg
Onions, mature	40 mg
Parsley	122 mg
Parsnips	50 mg
Peppers, sweet	6 mg
Peppers, hot	26 mg
Pickles, dill (1 small)	3 mg
Potato	11 mg
Pumpkin	24 mg
Radish (10)	9 mg
Rutabaga	92 mg
Sauerkraut	85 mg
Spinach	30 mg
Squash, summer	36 mg
Squash, winter	57 mg
Sweet potato	29 mg
Tomato, medium	8 mg
Tomato juice	17 mg
Tomato paste	71 mg
Turnip greens	105 mg
Turnips	51 mg
Vegetable juice cocktail	29 mg

There you have it. As I've been saying all along the dark-green, leafy vegetables provide the highest source of calcium, with kale (90 mg), dandelion greens (103 mg), turnip greens (105 mg), parsley (122 mg, but a cup of parsley is a lot of parsley), and chicory greens (180 mg) topping the list.

Oh, Nuts

Chopped nuts and seeds are rich in calcium and can easily be added to vegetables, cereals, yogurt, and salads.

NUTS AND SEEDS	CALCIUM
(mg of calcium in ½ cup, unless otherwise specified)	
Almonds	166 mg
Brazil nuts	130 mg
Cashews, dry roasted	26 mg
Chestnuts, raw, peeled	22 mg
Coconut, shredded	5 mg
Hazelnuts	141 mg
Macadamia nuts	47 mg
Pecans	40 mg
Pine nuts	16 mg
Pistachios	87 mg
Pumpkin and squash seeds	36 mg
Sesame seeds	702 mg
Sunflower seeds	87 mg
Walnuts, shelled	50 mg

As you can see, nuts and seeds, for the most part, provide high amounts of calcium and make great snacks, either on their own or sprinkled on top of other foods.

Don't Go Nuts with Nuts

Nuts do tend to be high in fat, so keep this in mind.

Legumes

These pod-borne vegetables, once considered "the poor man's meat" are loaded with nutrients and are fast becoming a popular, healthy mainstay in the American diet.

Legumes

Legumes are dried beans, peas, and lentils. They are veritable storehouses for valuable nutrients and are also a high source of protein. Unlike nuts, they are not high in fat. But both legumes and nuts are actually seeds, meaning that their small pods or shells contain enough nutrients to reproduce themselves and support new life until they can start getting additional nutrients from the soil. Here are a few you should know about:

Calcium Interactions

The calcium in legumes is only half as available as the calcium in milk.

Peas, pinto beans, and **navy beans** are high in **phytates**, which interfere with absorption.

LEGUMES	CALCIUM
(mg of calcium in 1 cup, cooked, unless otherwise noted)	
Black beans, cooked	46 mg
Black-eyed peas, cooked	40 mg
Fava beans, cooked	61 mg
Garbanzo beans, cooked	80 mg
Green peas	36 mg
Kidney beans, cooked	50 mg
Lentils, cooked	38 mg
Lima beans, cooked	32 mg
Peanuts, raw	104 mg
Peas, split, cooked	22 mg
Pinto beans, cooked	82 mg
Soybeans, cooked	175 mg

Fish and Shellfish

They are an excellent source of protein, but unlike meat and poultry, are quite low in calories, fat, and cholesterol, except for shrimp, which has 166 mg of cholesterol per three ounces. They are also good sources of vitamin B12, iodine, phosphorus, selenium, and zinc.

Tempeh	**111 mg**
Tofu (firm, processed with calcium carbonate)	**204 mg**

FISH, SHELLFISH	CALCIUM
(amount of calcium in 3 ounces, unless otherwise specified)	
Anchovy, in oil, drained (5)	**46 mg**
Bass, sea	**8.5 mg**
Bluefish	**6 mg**
Carp	**35 mg**
Caviar, black and red (1 tbsp)	**42 mg**
Clams (9 large)	**83 mg**
Cod	**13 mg**
Crab	**39 mg**
Flounder and sole	**15 mg**
Haddock	**28 mg**
Halibut	**40 mg**
Lobster	**26 mg**
Mackerel	**10 mg**
Oysters (6 medium)	**38 mg**
Perch	**91 mg**
Pike	**48 mg**
Salmon	**10 mg**
Salmon, canned with bones	**200 mg**
Sardines, canned with bones	**262 mg**
Scallops	**21 mg**
Shrimp	**44 mg**
Smelt	**51 mg**
Snails	**48 mg**
Snapper	**27 mg**

Swordfish	**4 mg**
Trout	**36 mg**
Tuna, bluefin	**6.8 mg**
Whitefish	**22 mg**

Grains

In most parts of the world, grain products—flour, cereal, bread, and pasta—are the primary sources of food. According to the *UC Berkeley Wellness Letter Book,* 50% of the world's calories come from grains. They contribute much to the other half of the world's calories (the non-grain half), since grain is fed to the animals from which we get meat, eggs, and dairy products. Whole grains provide the best source of complex carbohydrates, and many nutritionists recommend that we get from 55 to 60% of our calorie intake from carbohydrates. Not all grains come from the same botanical family. True grains—rice, wheat, oats, rye, millet, triticale, and barley—belong to the grass family *gramineae.* Other grains like amaranth, quinoa, and buckwheat belong to a different family, but they all have a kernel, defined as an edible seed. Many grains are milled and sometimes refined before we eat them. Refined grains are often enriched, to put back some of the nutrients that have been lost in the refining process, but they are still not as good for us as whole grains. I suggest you eat whole-grain products whenever possible. Here's the low-down on the calcium content in mg per cup of a variety of grains:

> **The Goodness of Grains**
>
> Whole grains are rich in complex carbohydrates and soluble fiber (which lowers cholesterol) and insoluble fiber (which prevents constipation). They also provide lots of the B vitamins (riboflavin, thiamine, and niacin), vitamin E, iron, zinc, selenium, magnesium, and, you guessed it, calcium.

GRAINS
(amount of calcium per cup)

Amaranth	**298 mg**
Barley, scotch or pot	**68 mg**
Buckwheat, groats	**28 mg**
Bulgur	**49 mg**

Cornmeal, whole grain	7.3 mg
Millet	16 mg
Oats	84 mg
Pasta, couscous	42 mg
Pasta, macaroni, enriched	19 mg
Pasta, whole-wheat spiral	42 mg
Pasta, spaghetti, enriched	10 mg
Pasta, spaghetti, whole wheat	23 mg
Rice, brown	64 mg
Rice, white, enriched	17 mg
Rice, wild	30 mg
Quinoa	102 mg

BREADS

Bagel, enriched	66 mg
English muffin, enriched	99 mg
English muffin, whole wheat	175 mg
French, enriched	19 mg
Mixed seven-grain	24 mg
Pita, enriched	24 mg
Pumpernickel	27 mg
Rye	23 mg
White, enriched	20 mg
Whole wheat	23 mg

THE NOT SO GOOD

Please don't get me wrong here. When I talk about the not-so-good foods—meats, poultry, and some fats and oils—it is not that the foods themselves are not good. Quite the contrary, in many cases. It is just that too much protein can make calcium absorption difficult, and too much saturated fat can lead to heart problems and obesity. I'll tell you all about what to eat with what in Chapters 9 and 10, but for now, here is a quick rundown on the amount of calcium in some of the major foods in these food groups.

Red Meat

Red meat is one of the major sources of fat and cholesterol (20 to 25 mg of cholesterol per ounce, whether fatty or lean meat) in the American diet. Try to eat meat in moderation.

MEAT	CALCIUM
(the amount of calcium in 1 pound, unless otherwise specified; remember that the recommended portion size is only 4 ounces, so divide these figures by 4 to see how much calcium there will be in a 4-ounce portion)	
Beef, chuck roast	32 mg
Beef, corned, brisket	30 mg
Beef, flank steak	22 mg
Beef, ground, lean	36 mg
Beef, ground, regular	40 mg
Beef liver	24 mg
Beef, porterhouse steak	29 mg
Beef, rib roast	39 mg
Beef, short ribs	41 mg
Beef, sirloin steak	34 mg
Beef, T-bone steak	30 mg
Beef, tenderloin	30 mg
Lamb, leg	0.39 mg
Lamb chops	35 mg
Lamb, liver	45 mg
Lamb, shoulder	35 mg
Pork, bacon	34 mg
Pork, Canadian bacon	36 mg
Pork, ham	0.32 mg
Pork, leg	25 mg
Pork, loin chop (1 chop)	7 mg
Pork, shoulder	24 mg
Pork, spareribs	19 mg

Veal, breast	39 mg
Veal cutlet	41 mg
Veal, liver	36 mg
Veal, rib roast	38 mg
Veal, rump roast	38 mg
Veal, sweetbreads	41 mg

POULTRY

Chicken, dark meat, no skin	54 mg
Chicken, white meat, no skin	40 mg
Chicken liver (1)	3 mg
Cornish game hen	38 mg
Duck, domesticated	48 mg
Goose, domesticated	53 mg
Turkey, dark meat	78 mg
Turkey, white meat	57 mg

WILD GAME

Rabbit	72 mg
Venison	45 mg
Pheasant (13 ounces)	46 mg
Quail (14 ounces)	52 mg

Meat and Poultry Tips

Always trim external fat from red meat and remove skin from poultry. Both beef and poultry are about 21% protein by weight.

Fats and Oils

Fats and oils are present in almost all foods. Butter, lard, and suet come from animals, while oils that we use for cooking and salads, as well as margarine, come from nuts, seeds, fruits (such as olives), and vegetables. Fats and oils are part of a group of substances called lipids, and lipids are biological chemicals that do not dissolve in water. The difference between a fat and an oil is that at room temperature, fats are solid while oils are liquid, but both are still fats. As you know, there is good fat and not-so-good fat. All fats and oils are made up of fatty acids, and fatty acids are made up of saturated fat and unsaturated fat, which refers to the degree to which a fatty acid is saturated by hydrogen atoms. Unsaturated fat is further divided into monounsaturated fat and polyunsaturated fat, the former having a slight edge over the latter in that it is more stable and less likely to be broken down by harmful oxidation, which can increase the risk of heart disease. It is always a good idea to keep the fats in your diet to a minimum, but it is especially important to reduce the amount of saturated fats (those found in animal fats and tropical oils such as coconut and palm oils). Cholesterol, a fatty substance, is found in foods derived from animals too, but cholesterol is not found in any plant-based oils. The important fact to remember here is that unsaturated vegetable oil will lower total and LDL (bad) cholesterol while maintaining or even increasing levels of HDL (good) cholesterol. Trans fats and saturated fats both raise your cholesterol level, but trans fats also lower your HDL. This is why trans fats are even worse for you than saturated fats.

There is virtually no calcium in the fats and oils we use, except for trace amounts in butter (3.37 mg per tablespoon), margarine (4.23 mg per tablespoon), olive oil (0.02 mg per tablespoon), peanut oil (0.01 mg per tablespoon), soybean oil (0.01 mg per tablespoon), and sunflower oil (0.03 per tablespoon).

Where do we stand, so far? It should be clear by now that milk, yogurt, and cheese (especially hard cheese) are excellent sources of calcium. Swiss

---

Trans Fats

To make vegetable oils become solid and shelf stable at room temperature—for margarine, vegetable shortening, cookies, chips, and crackers—manufacturers add hydrogen to them. This hydrogenation changes unsaturated fatty acids into saturated fatty acids called "trans fats," and these tend to increase bad blood cholesterol levels (LDL) while lowering good blood cholesterol levels (HDL). Since July 2003, the FDA has required that all food labels include the amount of trans fats in a product.

chard, kale, turnip greens, broccoli, canned sardines, canned salmon eaten with their soft bones, and firm tofu (processed with calcium carbonate) are, too. There are also excellent sources of nondairy calcium-fortified products on the market now. These include fortified juices such as grapefruit and orange juice, some mineral waters, breads, cereals, cheeses, and tofu. I suggest you buy calcium-fortified products whenever possible. Always check the label to see how much calcium is actually in the product. Remember, if the label says the product provides 30% of your daily calcium needs, you just add a "0" to figure out how much calcium (300 mg) is in this particular product.

THE TERRIBLE

Now I'm going to talk briefly about the foods and substances that you should avoid like the plague, or at least use only in moderation. We all know what they are: caffeine, tobacco (smoking), alcohol (too much of it), salt, refined sugar, and of course, too much protein in your diet. The real killers when it comes to calcium absorption are alcohol and tobacco. We'll get to those, but let's start with caffeine.

CAFFEINE

Like tobacco and alcohol, caffeine is an anti-nutrient. Instead of providing the body with nutrition, anti-nutrients rob the body and bones of the good nutrients they already have. Caffeine is a naturally occurring substance found in the leaves, fruits, or seeds of sixty-three different plants, including coffee beans, tea leaves, cola nuts, and cocoa beans. It is actually an organic compound with alkaline properties, and it belongs to the chemical family known as *methylxanthines*. What this all means is that even though it occurs naturally in many beverages, it is really a chemical that has druglike effects on the body. We all know how addictive caffeine can be. Caffeine acts as a stimulant on the heart and brain. That is why so many of us need a cup of coffee to wake up in the morning, or why we drink cola all day to keep going. *Caffeinism* is actually a disease caused by the nervousness and sleepless-ness brought on by consuming too much caffeine.

Research suggests that caffeine increases the amount of calcium we lose in the urine, and therein lies the problem. Also, most of us tend to replace the milk we once drank with coffee, tea, and cola, so we not only lose the additional calcium we would have been getting from milk, we leach out the calcium we already have through the urine, because of the increase in caffeine. Several studies have shown that caffeine and calcium don't go well together. The most recent study was published in 1990 in the *American Journal of Clinical Nutrition,* and it was conducted by Dr. Robert Heaney and his colleagues at Creighton University in Nebraska. Dr. Heaney and his research team gave sixteen women 400 mg of

Calcium Loss

We lose between 100 to 250 mg of calcium every day through the kidneys into the urine. Caffeine increases that loss.

Caffeine in Coffee

A cup of regular coffee is 5 ounces. A mug usually holds 10 ounces. Keep this in mind when figuring out how much caffeine you consume each day.

caffeine per day for nineteen days. These women also had calcium intakes of 600 mg or more per day, and they took a multivitamin to provide vitamin D. The doctors measured the amount of calcium lost in the urine while the women took the caffeine for twelve days. What did they find? They found that 400 mg of caffeine per day did not appear to be harmful, if the women were getting at least 600 mg of calcium in their diet each day. They also found that the loss of calcium in the urine probably only occurred for three hours after taking the caffeine and did not continue for the rest of the day. What is the bottom line here? Try to limit your caffeine intake to 400 mg per day, and make sure you are getting at the very least 600 mg of calcium plus vitamin D every day. Just how much caffeine is in coffee, tea, and cola? A cup of regular coffee (five ounces) contains two to three times more caffeine than tea or cola. Try not to have more than two to three servings of high-caffeine drinks a day, and as long as you are getting enough calcium in your diet, there should be nothing to worry about. Here's a list from the U.S. Food and Drug Administration and the National Soft Drink Association that should give you a pretty good idea of just how much caffeine there is in what you drink. As you can see, two mugs of regular drip coffee per day (20 ounces of coffee) could give you as much as 600 mg of caffeine, so keep an eye on your coffee consumption, try to switch to decaf, or limit yourself to two ordinary five-ounce cups a day, and you should be fine. If you decide to switch from regular coffee to decaf, as many of my patients have, you can avoid withdrawal symptoms by cutting back gradually. If you are addicted to caffeine and you simply give it up, you might get headaches for a few days. For some people, a few days of headaches are easier to deal with than gradual withdrawal. The stunning statistic as far as I'm concerned is that you can get as much as 150 mg of caffeine in a regular five-ounce cup of regular coffee (and remember, that's a pretty small cup), compared with 2 to 6 mg in a five-ounce cup of decaffeinated coffee. I think it makes a lot of sense to switch to decaf, and that's what I suggest to people when they ask for my advice. Make the switch and you'll be eliminating much of the calcium-leaching caffeine from your diet with this one simple change.

Caffeine Content in Various Beverages

COFFEE (five ounces)	CAFFEINE
Drip	110–150 mg
Percolated	64–124 mg
Instant	40–108 mg
Decaffeinated	2–5 mg
Instant decaffeinated	2 mg
TEA (five ounces, leaves or bag)	
One-minute brew time	9–33 mg
Three-minute brew time	20–46 mg
Five-minute brew time	20–50 mg
Instant tea (five ounces)	12–28 mg
Iced tea (twelve ounces)	22–36 mg
Cocoa (five ounces)	4 mg
Chocolate milk (eight ounces)	5 mg
SOFT DRINKS	
Cocoa-Cola	46.5 mg
Dr. Pepper	39.6 mg
Pepsi-Cola	38.4
RC Cola	36 mg
Mountain Dew	54 mg
Root Beer	0 mg

Tobacco (Smoking)

If you are a smoker, you are probably tired of hearing how bad it is for you. You know it can cause lung cancer, emphysema, bronchitis, and heart disease, but did you know that it greatly increases your risk of developing osteoporosis? How? Smoking, for women, apparently poisons the ovaries and reduces the effectiveness of the estrogen they produce. Here is what recent studies have shown about the effect of smoking in premenopausal women.

Smoking:

1. Reduces the amount of estrogen produced in the ovaries
2. Causes the estrogen that has been produced to be changed in the liver, making it useless
3. Causes premature menopause, along with total shutdown of the ovaries so that they become useless in the estrogen-production department

All of this leads to unnecessary, premature bone loss. In the Nurses Health Study of 116,229 women over a period of twelve years, women who smoked had a 30% greater risk of hip fracture than women who didn't. And the more a woman smokes, the greater her risk. Women who smoke more than twenty-five cigarettes a day increase their risk of hip fracture by 60%.

For postmenopausal women who smoke, the picture is not so pretty, either. Postmenopausal women produce very little estrogen, and these low levels of estrogen appear to be similar in smoking and nonsmoking postmenopausal women. But for those postmenopausal women on hormone replacement therapy (HRT) who are smokers, the effect of estrogen in the pill is not able to affect or protect their bones. This is because just as for premenopausal women, smoking causes the liver to change the estrogen into an undesirable form called 2-hydroxyestrone. This is a useless form of estrogen that is quickly eliminated by the body. A 1992 study in the *Annals of Internal Medicine* found that estrogen appeared to protect postmenopausal women taking HRT from hip fracture. This was not the case for those women who were smokers.

Is there a lesson here? Sure. The lesson is that smoking, which is bad for us at any age, is really bad as we begin to get older. It is especially dangerous for women when it comes to osteoporosis, because it interferes with the benefits of estrogen. If you are a smoker, stop. Just do it. There are all kinds of programs to help you out, and stopping is one of the best things you can possibly do for your bone health and your health in general.

Alcohol

Alcohol is the third of the anti-nutrients. It is packed with empty calories, and people who drink a lot tend to not eat a balanced diet to get the nutrition they need from healthy foods, so they end up being deficient in all kinds of important vitamins and minerals. Here are some of the things excessive alcohol can do:

1. It can decrease the absorption of calcium by damaging the intestinal tract.
2. It can damage the liver so that the liver can't make the vitamin D that the body needs to absorb calcium.
3. It can damage the pancreas, which is the organ that gives us the enzymes necessary to digest food, so that we can't absorb vitamin D and calcium and other important nutrients.

There is evidence suggesting that alcohol poisons the osteoblasts (bone builders) and so has a direct effect on bone itself. Also, people who have had too much to drink fall more easily than others, and this contributes to broken hips, spines, and wrists in people who are already at high risk of having osteoporosis. It is true that one study suggested that no more than two glasses of red wine a day may be healthy for postmenopausal women, but as with so much in life, the trick is moderation. I'm not suggesting that we all become teetotalers, but it is so important to try to keep drinking under control. It is important for your bones, your general health, and your relationships. If you think you might have a problem, be reassured that there is help everywhere. Alcoholics Anonymous groups exist in almost every city in the country, and your local ministers, priests, and rabbis are always available for counseling. Because alcohol is so addictive, it is one of those things that can sneak up on you. There is no shame in that. The important thing is to try to control the

Alcohol and Bones

Alcohol can poison our osteoblasts (the bone builders), thereby directly affecting bone health.

addiction before it starts to eat away at your bones, your health, and your relationships with the people you love and respect.

Salt

Throw away the saltshaker. That's my advice, and I'll tell you why. Even though some salt is essential to our health, the National Research Council suggests that we limit our salt intake to 2,300 mg (about one teaspoon) per day. Most of the salt in our diet comes from processed foods, not from the salt we add to the food we eat. Because we get too much salt from processed foods, it is a good idea not to add more to any of the fresh foods in our diet. It is important that we limit our salt intake because too much salt can cause us to lose calcium and other important vitamins and minerals through our urine. In fact, several studies have shown that an intake of more than 3,000 mg of salt a day increases urinary loss of calcium, increasing the risk of bone loss. One study of postmenopausal women conducted at the University of Western Australia in 1995 showed that when women cut their salt intake in half (down to about 1,200 mg per day), their reduction of bone loss is what it would have been had they increased the calcium in their diet by 900 mg per day. There is a big difference between the kind of salt we buy in the supermarket and sea salt, which comes from evaporated seawater. Commercial supermarket salt, taken from old mines, is high in sodium-based additives such as yellow prussiate of soda and sodium silico aluminate, as well as potassium iodide and additives that make the salt look good but are questionable when it comes to human health. Sea salt has no additives, so it is much healthier—that is, if you feel you must use salt at all.

Cut down on processed foods (generally speaking, those foods that require a package label), and always read the label on the processed foods you do buy. There are sodium salts in any ingredient containing the word sodium or salt. Watch out for words like sodium propionate, bicarbonate of soda, sodium citrate, monosodium glutamate, sodium nitrate, sodium nitrite, sodium bisulfite, sodium benzoate, sodium

> **Salt**
>
> **Table salt, known as sodium chloride, can increase the amount of calcium lost in the urine dramatically. Try to limit salt to 2,000 mg per day.**

stearoyl lactylate, and sodium caseinate. These are all sodium-based commercial food additives.

Try to stay away from canned foods and fast foods, because they are loaded with salt. One cup of canned tomato sauce has 1,498 mg sodium, one cup of canned pork and beans has 2,130 mg sodium, a cup of canned split-pea soup has 1,956 mg sodium, four slices of bacon have 548 mg sodium, three ounces of ham has 1,114 mg sodium, a slice of pizza can have 600 mg sodium, and smoked fish can have up to 5,000 mg sodium. Be aware that processed foods, which make up more than 80% of our diet, are very high in salt. Read the labels carefully, and if possible, as I suggested before, never touch the saltshaker.

Refined Sugar

Sugars are simple carbohydrates. Glucose and fructose come from fruits and some vegetables, lactose is the sugar in milk, and sucrose comes from cane or beet sugar. Most of the simple carbohydrates we Americans consume are those that have been added to processed foods such as cookies, cakes, and soft drinks. These added sugars, especially sucrose, account for 16% of all the calories in our diet, according to the *UC Berkeley Wellness Letter Book*. Twenty years ago, added sugars only contributed 11% of our calories. The trouble with this is that most processed foods high in added sugar give us a lot of "empty calories," without providing many of the important nutrients we need to stay healthy. The best way to get your simple carbohydrates (sugars) is from fruits, fruit juices, and low-fat milk, because these foods are also rich in other important nutrients. Too much refined sugar in your diet can make you more susceptible to developing diabetes, and we all know that excess sugar contributes to obesity, which is rising at an alarming rate in this country. My advice is to stay away from refined sugars as much as possible. Instead, replace them with fresh fruits, vegetables, low-fat milk, and other high-calcium foods.

PROTEIN

Protein is good for us. Everybody knows that. But too much protein, especially animal protein, can be bad for us, especially when it comes to calcium absorption. Too much protein actually washes out calcium from the body.

How much is too much? The recommended daily allowance is 44 grams per day for women, and 56 grams per day for men. Since one four-ounce serving of meat contains 35 grams of protein, you can see how easy it is to go over the limit. We need protein to help form collagen, and we also need vitamin C to stimulate the enzymes that form the collagen and connective tissue. Protein is found in meats, poultry, fish, eggs, nuts, seeds, and some grains. If you cut down on animal sources of protein, especially red meat, and keep your portions small (no more than four ounces of meat at a meal), you can greatly reduce your protein intake, retaining more of the calcium you eat and cutting your risk of heart disease, as well. Just for the record, a one-pound porterhouse steak has a whopping 78.8 grams of protein. Now that's food for thought.

> **Protein**
>
> Most Americans eat more than 100 grams of protein per day. That's about twice the recommended daily allowance.

> **Vegetarians**
>
> Vegetarians have a much lower risk of osteoporosis than people who eat meat. Their initial bone is similar to non-vegetarians but once bone loss starts the **rate of loss is much slower** than in non-vegetarians.

WHAT DOES THIS HAVE TO DO WITH ME?

You'll notice a lot of *don't*s and *no*'s and such in this chapter, but don't get discouraged. Sticking with a diet that is good for your bones is not all that difficult, and need not feel restrictive. We'll go into this in detail in the next two chapters, but now let me give you a quick summary of my experience about what really works when it comes to helping people eat right for maximum bone health.

Just to be on the safe side, it wouldn't be a bad idea to take one to two 500 mg tablets of calcium with vitamin D a day also. This is especially important if you live in a climate where you can't count on at least ten minutes of direct sunlight on a daily basis. And do pay special attention to tip number 10, below. Eating in a relaxed environment and chewing your food well can make a big difference in how well your body is able to absorb the valuable nutrients you give it.

Ten Diet Tips for Healthy Bones

1. **Reduce the animal protein** in your diet. Eat no more than four ounces of red meat and poultry (the size of the palm of your hand) per day if you are a woman, or six ounces if you are a man.
2. **Reduce the salt** in your diet. Try to keep it to 2,000 mg per day. Throw away the saltshaker.
3. **Reduce foods high in saturated fat.**
4. **Reduce alcohol intake.** Limit yourself to two drinks per day.
5. **Stop smoking.**
6. **Reduce caffeine.** Switch from regular to decaffeinated coffee.
7. **Increase vegetables, fruits, legumes, beans, and whole grains,** especially green, leafy vegetables.
8. **Increase calcium-rich foods.**
9. **Increase the amount of water your drink** to at least ten eight-ounce glasses per day.
10. **Eat in a relaxed setting and chew your food slowly and well.**

CHAPTER NINE

THE 14-DAY, HEALTHY, HIGH-CALCIUM DIET

THE 7-DAY, HEALTHY, HIGH-CALCIUM DIET FOR THE LACTOSE-INTOLERANT

THE 7-DAY, HEALTHY, HIGH-CALCIUM DIET FOR VEGETARIANS

Healthy Eating Plans to Help You Maximize Calcium Absorption—Naturally—from the Foods You Eat

Just like the seasons, diets come and go. At one time or another, most of us have tried to take off a few pounds, hoping to emerge with a whole new body after just a few weeks on, say, a low-fat diet, a high-fiber diet, a liquid diet, a grapefruit diet, or one of those fancy food-combining or food-cycling diets. Even though we may see some positive results in the short run, the effects of these food diets usually wear off after a few months, and many of us end up gaining back more weight than we lost in the first place.

My Healthy, High-Calcium Diet is not based on any fad. It is designed to show you precisely how to get at least 1,500 mg of calcium every day the natural, healthy way, through the foods you eat. New research suggests that a high-calcium diet can lead to weight loss. According to a 1999 report from the Federation of American Societies for Experimental Biology, a high-calcium diet may help decrease body fat, at least among college-age women who routinely eat fewer than 1,900 calories a day. Among these women, those who got at least 780 mg of calcium daily showed no increase in body fat during the two-year study. In fact, those who got 1,000 mg of calcium daily actually lost an average of six pounds each. Women eating the same number of calories but little calcium, meanwhile, had increases in body fat.

You may indeed find that you shed a few pounds on my diet, but that is not its primary goal. My diet is designed to give you the best nutrition possible while also maximizing your calcium intake, in order to help ward off the risk of osteoporosis.

Before we get to the diet itself, let's just brush up on what healthy nutrition is all about in the first place. Every *body* needs energy, and energy comes from three sources: carbohydrates, proteins, and fats. Their energy content is interchangeable—in other words, all of these sources provide energy. The difference between them is there are:

4 calories in a gram of carbohydrate
4 calories in a gram of protein
9 calories in a gram of fat
(By the way, 1 gram equals 1/28 ounce, or 1 ounce equals 28 grams)

Another difference between these nutrients is the speed at which they provide energy. Carbohydrates are the quickest to be metabolized, proteins are the second quickest, and fats are the slowest. They are all digested in the intestine, where (with a little help from fiber) they are broken down into their basic units:

Carbohydrates into sugars
Proteins into amino acids
Fats into fatty acids and glycerol

After they are broken down, the body uses these substances for growth, maintenance, and energy. When it comes to how much of each of these you need in your daily diet, most nutritionists agree with the latest recommendations from the American Dietetic Association:

Carbohydrates should provide 45 to 65% of your daily calories.
Protein should provide 5 to 20% of your daily calories.
Fat should be limited to less than 40% of your daily calories,
with the emphasis on the good fats—polyunsaturated and
monounsaturated—such as those found in vegetable oils.

Another way to look at this is that when it comes to the number of grams every day, a healthy, 2,000-calorie diet should contain approximately:

Carbohydrates:	**240 grams (960 calories)**
Protein	**60 grams (240 calories), although I feel that 45 grams for most women is adequate**
Fat:	**Less than 90 grams (810 calories)**
Fiber:	**30 grams (This tough, complex carbohydrate is only partially digested and provides bulk to help move feces through the intestine, moderates sugar and cholesterol levels, prevents diverticular disease, and eliminates cancer-causing bacteria from the intestine.)**

CALORIES

A calorie is simply a measure of energy. Foods contain calories that supply the body with energy when the food is broken down in the digestive system. This amazing phenomenon called "energy" allows the cells to perform all of their functions. This energy can be stored or used right away.

When the body takes in more energy than it needs—that is, when there are more calories in your roast beef and baked potato dinner than your body can use right away—your body stores those extra calories as fat, although some are stored as carbohydrates in the liver and muscle. The result—no surprise here—is that you gain weight. An extra 200 calories a day for ten days will probably cause you to gain at least a half a pound.

When you take in less energy (fewer calories) than your body needs, the body starts to use the carbohydrates stored in the liver and muscle to get its energy. This usually leads to quick, short-term weight loss, because these carbohydrates are metabolized quickly and water is excreted as they are metabolized. Soon, though, these carbohydrates are used up and the body turns to stored fat as its source of energy. Converting this fat into energy is a slower process, so after the initial spurt of weight loss the whole process starts to slow down. Fat can provide energy for a long time. Rarely does the body of a normally nourished person break down protein. If you were starving—that is, eating no food at all—protein would eventually start to break down and you would probably live for only eight to twelve weeks, not a pleasant thought at all.

Did you ever wonder how scientists figure out how many calories are in a given food? It's simple. They burn the food. That's right, they just put a sample of the food in an insulated, oxygen-filled, boxlike device called a *bomb calorimeter,* and surround it with water. Then they burn the sample completely in a procedure called *calorimetry*. When the food burns, the heat in the surrounding water increases the temperature of the water. The temperature increase indicates the number of calories in the food. If the temperature increases by 35 degrees, then the food contains 35 calories.

Each body is unique, and calorie requirements vary greatly depending on your gender, height, weight, physical activity, metabolic rate, and age. You can require anywhere from 1,000 to 4,000 calories a day. Generally speaking, though, here's what works in terms of the calories per day needed to maintain body weight for most people:

1,600 calories	**Young children, sedentary women, older adults**
2,000 calories	**Older children, active adult women, sedentary men**
2,400 calories	**Active adolescent boys and young men**

All of this is approximate, and it is important to remember that the body requires different amounts of calories at different times to maintain body weight. If you are doing a lot of exercise, especially aerobic exercise, you will need many more calories than if you spend the day at the computer, reading, watching TV, and chatting on the phone.

In Chapter 7, I discussed in detail the suggested amounts of various vitamins and minerals you need in your diet each day. You should refer to that chapter periodically to see just how many of the most important vitamins and minerals you'll be getting when you start to use one of the three diets listed in the title of this chapter:

○ The 14-Day, Healthy, High-Calcium Diet

○ The 7-Day, Healthy, High-Calcium Diet for the Lactose-Intolerant

○ The 7-Day, Healthy, High-Calcium Diet for Vegetarians

There is one more point I'd like to make before getting into the diets. I have tried to keep them simple. Busy people often don't have time to do much cooking, especially during the week. This is why I have recommended only easy-to-find, easy-to-use foods in my daily diets. Please note that when a recipe calls for tofu, I am usually referring to the firm tofu that has been processed with calcium carbonate. I realize that many of you may not be familiar with tofu, but don't dismiss it until you've tried it. It can be delicious and high in calcium when you use the firm variety I've just described. Also, you can drink as much coffee (preferably decaffeinated), tea, or water as you would like at any meal. Drink as much water as you can, at least ten eight-ounce glasses a day, if possible. In the Cookbook section (Section Four) you'll find a wide selection of delicious, high-calcium gourmet recipes that you can prepare when you have the time. Use them whenever you want in place of the simple-to-prepare foods I suggest in the daily menus for each of the diets. I have also included a small section called "High-Calcium Recipes for Kids," since the best time for building maximum bone strength is when we are young.

The 14-Day, Healthy, High-Calcium Diet

MENU FOR MONDAY (DAY 1)

BREAKFAST	CALCIUM (mg)	CALORIES
Yogurt parfait:		
1 cup plain, nonfat yogurt layered with	404	207
½ oz General Mills® Fiber-One	47	28
½ cup strawberries	11	23
2 tbsp raisins	5	54
2 slices whole-wheat toast	47	130
2 tsp margarine	3	67
Decaf coffee or tea		

SNACK		
1 apple	0	80

LUNCH		
Vegetable melt:		
½ cup broccoli	17	10
½ cup bok choy	37	5
½ cup brussels sprouts	18	19
½ cup carrots	17	28
Cover with:		
1 oz low-fat Swiss	272	51
1 oz low-fat cheddar	118	49
Microwave for about 1–2 minutes.		
Small baked sweet potato	23	95
8 oz 1% milk	300	102
Decaf coffee or tea		

SNACK		
2 rice cakes	2	70
2 tbsp peanut butter	17	187

DINNER	CALCIUM	CALORIES
6 cheese ravioli (DiGiorno®)	500	560
½ cup marinara sauce	23	85
1 cup broccoli rabe sauteed with garlic	53	33
Salad with lettuce, tomato, cucumber, celery	46	26
Decaf coffee or tea		

SNACK		
1 frozen fruit and juice bar	4	63

Total Calcium: 1,965 mg ○ **Total Calories: 1,970**

Basic Components

Calories	1,970		Minerals	
Protein	95 g		Boron	5 mcg
Carbohydrates	306 g		Calcium	1,965 mg
Dietary Fiber	35 g		Copper	1 mg
Total Fat	52 g		Magnesium	349 mg
Saturated Fat	17 g		Manganese	5 mg
			Phosphorus	1,967 mg
Vitamins			Sodium	2,731 mg
Vitamin B6	2 mg		Zinc	10 mg
Vitamin B12	4 mcg			
Vitamin C	317 mg			
Vitamin D	100 IU			
Folate	539 mcg			
Vitamin K	92 mcg			

MENU FOR TUESDAY (DAY 2)

BREAKFAST	CALCIUM (mg)	CALORIES
1 cup oatmeal cooked with	9	73
1 cup 1% milk sweetened with	300	110
1 tsp blackstrap molasses		
and cinnamon	59	16
1 small, sliced banana	5	75
1 slice whole-grain toast	24	65
1 tsp strawberry jam	0	17
Decaf coffee or tea		

SNACK		
8 fl oz Tropicana Tropical Fruit Smoothie®	15	147

LUNCH		
1 grilled portobello mushroom topped with	0	40
1 oz Swiss cheese, melted	298	97
1 cup sauteed spinach	245	41
Large tossed salad	46	26
1 cup amaranth topped with	75	182
2 oz peas	5	16
2 tsp chopped walnuts	3	32

SNACK		
1 pear	23	123
1 oz Brie	52	95
¼ cup almonds	64	142

DINNER		
4 oz baked perch breaded with	117	103
¼ cup crushed General Mills Total®		
cereal	188	21
1 cup steamed bok choy	158	21

	CALCIUM	CALORIES
½ cup steamed brown rice and chopped scallion	10	108
Decaf coffee or tea		

SNACK	CALCIUM	CALORIES
1 x 2 x 2.5–inch piece baklava	33	336
6 oz 1% milk	225	77

Total Calcium: 1,952 mg ○ **Total Calories: 1,960**

Basic Components

Calories 1,960	**Minerals**
Protein 91 g	Boron 4 mcg
Carbohydrates 258 g	Calcium 1,952 mg
Dietary Fiber 36 g	Copper 3 mg
Total Fat 67 g	Magnesium 653 mg
Saturated Fat 25 g	Manganese 6 mg
	Phosphorus 1,709 mg
Vitamins	Sodium 1,284 mg
Vitamin B6 3 mg	Zinc 13 mg
Vitamin B12 3 mcg	
Vitamin C 133 mg	
Vitamin D 216 IU	
Folate 685 mcg	
Vitamin K 18 mcg	

MENU FOR WEDNESDAY (DAY 3)

BREAKFAST	CALCIUM (mg)	CALORIES
Swiss cheese omelette:		
2 eggs	49	149
2 oz low-fat Swiss cheese	597	194
8 oz fortified orange juice	350	110
2 slices whole-grain toast	47	130
2 tsp apricot jam	3	32
Decaf coffee or tea		

SNACK		
1 peach	5	42
3 celery sticks	32	13

LUNCH		
4 oz canned salmon with	282	160
2 tbsp chopped onion	4	8
1 tbsp low-fat mayo	1	50
½ cup sliced cucumber	7	7
1 Roma tomato	3	13
½ cup lettuce	10	4
1 scallion	11	5
2 Wasa® crackers	10	48
Decaf coffee or tea		

SNACK		
1 cup Breyers Black Cherries Jubilee®		
yogurt	200	120

DINNER		
4 oz grilled lamb chops	15	213
1 cup steamed spinach	86	22
1 cup romaine lettuce with	46	26
Sliced peppers	3	10
Carrots	13	22

Radishes	9	6
Baked potato topped with	17	188
2 tbsp Breakstone's® low-fat sour cream	50	47
1 tbsp chives	2	1
Decaf coffee or tea		

SNACK

1-oz wedge of Swiss cheese	272	107
1-oz wedge of Havarti	191	105
2 Wasa® crackers	10	48
1 pear	18	98

Total Calcium: 2,344 mg ○ **Total Calories: 1,975**

Basic Components

Calories 1,975	Minerals
Protein 132 g	Boron 4 mcg
Carbohydrates 215 g	Calcium 2,344 mg
Dietary Fiber 26 g	Copper 2 mg
Total Fat 69 g	Magnesium 316 mg
Saturated Fat 32 g	Manganese 4 mg
	Phosphorus 2,159 mg
Vitamins	Sodium 1,646 mg
Vitamin B6 3 mg	Zinc 16 mg
Vitamin B12 11 mcg	
Vitamin C 276 mg	
Vitamin D 321 IU	
Folate 454 mcg	
Vitamin K 78 mcg	

MENU FOR THURSDAY (DAY 4)

BREAKFAST	CALCIUM (mg)	CALORIES
Decaf café latte:		
4 oz coffee + 4 oz hot, low-fat milk	137	50
¾ cup fortified Total® cereal	945	92
½ cup low-fat milk	137	50
½ cup strawberries	12	25
1 whole-wheat English muffin	175	134
1 tbsp apricot preserves	4	48

SNACK		
2 Wasa® crackers	10	48
1 tbsp peanut butter	9	94
8 oz 1% milk	279	95

LUNCH		
3 oz store-bought broccoli and		
cheddar quiche	196	272
1 cup cream of broccoli soup	39	82
4 oz spinach salad	46	108
2 oz French bread	44	153
2 tsp margarine	3	34

SNACK		
Baked apple	12	102
¼ cup fat-free half and half	80	40

DINNER		
4 oz grilled wild salmon	17	206
1 med. baked potato topped with	17	188
3 oz yogurt and chives	159	55
1 cup steamed turnip greens	197	29

SNACK	CALCIUM	CALORIES
2 oatmeal cookies	10	85
8 oz 1% milk	300	102

Total Calcium: 2,826 mg   ⭘   **Total Calories: 2,091**

Basic Components

Calories 2,091	Minerals
Protein 102 g	Boron 7 mcg
Carbohydrates 287 g	Calcium 2,826 mg
Dietary Fiber 33 g	Copper 2 mg
Total Fat 64 g	Magnesium 420 mg
Saturated Fat 21 g	Manganese 5 mg
	Phosphorus 1,754 mg
Vitamins	Sodium 2,571 mg
Vitamin B6 5 mg	Zinc 23 mg
Vitamin B12 12 mcg	
Vitamin C 200 mg	
Vitamin D 642 IU	
Folate 877 mcg	
Vitamin K 33 mcg	

MENU FOR FRIDAY (DAY 5)

BREAKFAST	**CALCIUM (mg)**	**CALORIES**
Smoothie:		
½ cup milk	150	55
1 tbsp molasses	176	48
1 cup blackberries	46	75
½ cup diced banana	5	69
¼ cup vanilla low-fat yogurt	210	105

Mix in blender until thoroughly combined.

SNACK		
2 Wasa® crackers	10	48
1 tbsp almond butter	43	101
1 tbsp strawberry preserves	0	50

LUNCH		
Omelette:		
2 eggs	49	149
1 oz Swiss cheese	298	97
¼ cup green pepper strips	2	6
Salad:		
½ cup watercress	20	2
½ cup endive	9	8
2 tbsp oil and vinegar	9	139
2 slices whole-grain bread	47	130

SNACK		
½ cup blueberries	4	41
¼ cup fat-free half and half	80	40

DINNER		
4 oz broiled fillet of sole with	20	133
1 tbsp lemon juice	1	4
1 tsp butter	2	67
1 cup steamed broccoli sprinkled with	34	20

1 tsp sesame seeds	3	15
1 cup steamed bok choy	158	20
½ cup brown rice	10	108
1 cup tossed salad	46	26

SNACK

4 oz frozen yogurt	180	119
1 tsp toasted coconut	2	34
2 tbsp hot fudge	60	140
2 tbsp chopped walnuts	9	95
½ cup sliced banana	5	69

Total Calcium: 1,690 mg   **Total Calories: 2,011**

Basic Components

Calories 2,011	**Minerals**
Protein 95 g	Boron 3 mcg
Carbohydrates 251 g	Calcium 1,690 mg
Dietary Fiber 31 g	Copper 2 mg
Total Fat 76 g	Magnesium 476 mg
Saturated Fat 24 g	Manganese 7 mg
	Phosphorus 1,624 mg
Vitamins	Sodium 1,113 mg
Vitamin B6 3 mg	Zinc 10 mg
Vitamin B12 5 mcg	
Vitamin C 225 mg	
Vitamin D 177 IU	
Folate 480 mcg	
Vitamin K 53 mcg	

MENU FOR SATURDAY (DAY 6)

BREAKFAST	CALCIUM (mg)	CALORIES
1 oz Kellogg's All-Bran with Extra Fiber®		
cereal	118	54
4 oz 1% milk	150	55
2 tsp chopped almonds	11	24
8 oz calcium-fortified grapefruit juice	298	106
½ cup blackberries	23	37
1 whole-wheat English muffin	175	134
1 tbsp apricot jam	4	48
Decaf coffee or tea		

SNACK		
2 rice cakes	2	70
2 oz melted cheddar cheese	399	226

LUNCH		
Chef's salad (romaine, cucumber,		
tomato, onion) with	56	46
1 oz lean roast beef	1	50
1 oz low-fat Swiss	203	54
1 oz low-fat American	194	51
1 oz turkey	6	54
2 tbsp oil and vinegar	9	139

SNACK		
1 oz whole-wheat pretzels	8	103

DINNER		
Cheeseburger (3-oz burger)	8	282
1 oz low-fat American cheese	194	51
1 cup sauteed kale with garlic	90	34
1 cup sauteed collard greens with garlic	226	49
1 baked sweet potato	23	95

SNACK	CALCIUM	CALORIES
Peanut butter Smoothie:		
4 oz 1% milk	139	47
1 tbsp peanut butter	9	93
1½ tsp honey	1	32
1 small banana	6	93
Ice cubes		

Mix in blender until thoroughly combined.

Total Calcium: 2,353 mg ○ **Total Calories: 2,028**

Basic Components

Calories 2,028	**Minerals**
Protein 112 g	Boron 3 mcg
Carbohydrates 242 g	Calcium 2,353 mg
Dietary Fiber 43 g	Copper 2 mg
Total Fat 81 g	Magnesium 432 mg
Saturated Fat 30 g	Manganese 8 mg
	Phosphorus 1,875 mg
Vitamins	Sodium 2,333 mg
Vitamin B6 4 mg	Zinc 12 mg
Vitamin B12 9 mcg	
Vitamin C 286 mg	
Vitamin D IU 169 IU	
Folate 663 mcg	
Vitamin K 563 mcg	

MENU FOR SUNDAY (DAY 7)

BREAKFAST	CALCIUM (mg)	CALORIES
Grilled cheese sandwich:		
2 oz low-fat, low-sodium cheddar cheese	399	98
2 slices whole-grain bread	47	130
2 tsp margarine	3	67
8 oz fortified Tropicana® grapefruit juice	400	106

SNACK		
1 cup Dannon® blackberry yogurt	300	220

LUNCH		
Canned chili & beans	107	254
1 oz low-fat cheddar cheese		
(melted on chili)	199	49
1 cup steamed broccoli	34	20
1 cup steamed kale	94	36
1 oz corn chips	20	140
Decaf coffee or tea		

SNACK		
½ cantaloupe	40	100

DINNER		
6 oz canned black bean soup	38	104
3 oz turkey burger	21	193
Mixed-grain bun	41	113
Mixed sauteed vegetables including		
1 cup kale	94	36
1 cup mustard greens	104	21
½ cup amaranth with	182	75
2 tbsp sauteed mushrooms	5	6
Tossed salad	46	26

SNACK	CALCIUM	CALORIES
8 oz 1% milk	279	95
4 graham crackers	3	59

Total Calcium: 2,347 mg ○ **Total Calories: 2,056**

Basic Components

Calories 2,056	Minerals
Protein 118 g	Boron 4 mcg
Carbohydrates 287 g	Calcium 2,347 mg
Dietary Fiber 51 g	Copper 2 mg
Total Fat 59 g	Magnesium 486 mg
Saturated Fat 19 g	Manganese 5 mg
	Phosphorus 1,793 mg
Vitamins	Sodium 2,828 mg
Vitamin B6 2 mg	Zinc 15 mg
Vitamin B12 2 mcg	
Vitamin C 420 mg	
Vitamin D 143 IU	
Folate 623 mcg	
Vitamin K 9 mcg	

MENU FOR MONDAY (DAY 8)

BREAKFAST	CALCIUM (mg)	CALORIES
4 oz low-fat pineapple cottage cheese with	60	110
1 tbsp nonfat dry milk powder	57	15
2 slices whole-grain toast	47	130
2 tsp margarine	3	67
Decaf café latte (4 oz decaf coffee + 4 oz		
hot 1% milk)	150	55

SNACK		
1 apple	0	80
1 oz low-fat, low-sodium cheddar cheese	199	49

LUNCH		
Greek salad:		
2 cups romaine lettuce	40	16
¼ cup onion	8	15
1 tomato	3	13
½ cup cucumber	7	7
4 Calamata olives	5	42
3 anchovies	28	25
4 oz feta cheese	559	299
1 whole-wheat pita bread	10	170

SNACK		
½ grapefruit	20	60

DINNER		
4 oz grilled chicken breast (no skin)	17	187
½ cup buckwheat	6	77
1 tbsp chopped almonds	39	87
1 cup sauteed kale with garlic	94	36
1 cup sauteed collard greens with garlic	226	49
1 cup spinach salad	46	108
½ cup red pepper strips	5	16
2 tbsp oil and vinegar dressing	9	139

SNACK	CALCIUM	CALORIES
1 cup blueberries	9	81
½ cup fat-free sour cream	180	116

Total Calcium: 1,827 mg ○ **Total Calories: 2,051**

Basic Components

Calories 2,051	Minerals
Protein 119 g	Boron 1 mcg
Carbohydrates 232 g	Calcium 1,827 mg
Dietary Fiber 42 g	Copper 1 mg
Total Fat 80 g	Magnesium 309 mg
Saturated Fat 29 g	Manganese 6 mg
	Phosphorus 1,607 mg
Vitamins	Sodium 3,528 mg
Vitamin B6 3 mg	Zinc 10 mg
Vitamin B12 4 mcg	
Vitamin C 344 mg	
Vitamin D 92 IU	
Folate 575 mcg	
Vitamin K 11 mcg	

MENU FOR TUESDAY (DAY 9)

BREAKFAST	CALCIUM (mg)	CALORIES
2 oz Brie	104	189
3 dried figs	82	145
2 Wasa® whole-grain crackers	10	48
8 oz calcium-fortified Tropicana®		
orange juice	350	110
Decaf café latte (4 oz decaf coffee +		
4 oz hot 1% milk)	150	55

SNACK		
1 cup Breyers® low-fat		
apple cobbler yogurt	250	230

LUNCH		
1 can (3.25 oz) chopped sardines		
(with bones)	352	192
1 oz chopped onion	6	11
1 tsp lemon juice on	0	1
2 slices whole-grain toast	47	130

SNACK		
½ cup grapes	9	57
Graham crackers (8 rectangles)	7	118
1 tbsp almond butter	43	101

DINNER		
Chinese takeout:		
Steamed tofu (4 oz) with vegetables	397	86
½ cup bok choy	79	10
½ cup broccoli	17	10
½ cup pea pods	34	34
¼ cup carrots	12	18
½ cup brown rice	10	108
Decaf coffee or tea		

SNACK	CALCIUM	CALORIES
½ cup fruit salad	13	101
½ cup frozen yogurt	180	119
2 tbsp chocolate syrup	6	102

Total Calcium: 2,160 mg ○ **Total Calories: 1,974**

Basic Components

Calories 1,947	Minerals
Protein 86 g	Boron 2 mcg
Carbohydrates 293 g	Calcium 2,160 mg
Dietary Fiber 26 g	Copper 1 mg
Total Fat 55 g	Magnesium 359 mg
Saturated Fat 18 g	Manganese 5 mg
	Phosphorus 1,569 mg
Vitamins	Sodium 1,705 mg
Vitamin B6 2 mg	Zinc 8 mg
Vitamin B12 11 mcg	
Vitamin C 206 mg	
Vitamin D 304 IU	
Folate 318 mcg	
Vitamin K 15 mcg	

MENU FOR WEDNESDAY (DAY 10)

BREAKFAST	CALCIUM (mg)	CALORIES
8 oz low-fat vanilla yogurt	389	194
1 slice whole-grain toast	57	158
½ cup blackberries	23	37

SNACK		
2 celery stalks stuffed with	32	13
½ cup ricotta cheese topped with	337	171
1 tsp sesame seeds	30	17

LUNCH		
Grilled cheese sandwich:		
2 oz low-fat American cheese	388	102
1 oz low-fat cheddar cheese on	199	49
2 slices whole-grain bread with	47	130
2 tsp margarine	3	67
1 cup mesclun salad	46	26
2 tbsp oil and vinegar	0	119
1 orange	56	64

SNACK		
2 cups popcorn	2	110

DINNER		
Italian takeout:		
8 oz eggplant parmesan (baked)	420	366
1 tbsp low-sodium Parmesan cheese	86	29
1 cup tossed salad	46	26
1 tbsp Italian dressing	1	69
1 cup escarole sauteed with garlic	26	9

SNACK	CALCIUM	CALORIES
8 oz 1% milk	300	102
3-oz slice cheesecake	41	257

Total Calcium: 2,539 mg ◯ **Total Calories: 2,133**

Basic Components

Calories 2,133	**Minerals**
Protein 99 g	Boron 6 mcg
Carbohydrates 205 g	Calcium 2,539 mg
Dietary Fiber 29 g	Copper 1 mg
Total Fat 108 g	Magnesium 358 mg
Saturated Fat 39 g	Manganese 4 mg
	Phosphorus 2,257 mg
Vitamins	Sodium 3,310 mg
Vitamin B6 1 mg	Zinc 13 mg
Vitamin B12 4 mcg	
Vitamin C 167 mg	
Vitamin D 107 IU	
Folate 559 mcg	
Vitamin K 146 mcg	

MENU FOR THURSDAY (DAY 11)

BREAKFAST	CALCIUM (mg)	CALORIES
Frittata:		
2 eggs	51	183
1 oz low-fat Swiss	298	97
1 oz low-fat cheddar	199	49
½ cup broccoli	9	5
8 oz calcium-fortified orange juice	241	76
café latte (4 oz decaf coffee +		
4 oz hot 1% milk)	150	55

SNACK		
12 baby carrots	28	46
3 dried figs	82	145

LUNCH		
2 oz turkey	12	107
2 oz low-fat Swiss cheese on	597	194
2 slices whole-grain bread with	47	130
½ cup alfalfa sprouts	5	4
1 tomato	3	13
1 tsp mustard	0	5
½ cup coleslaw	13	8

SNACK		
1 peach	5	42

DINNER		
1 4-oz can sardines (with bones) over	433	236
1 cup tossed salad	46	26
1 small baked potato with	14	150
¼ cup yogurt and chives	115	40
1 cup steamed collard greens	52	11

SNACK	CALCIUM	CALORIES
Baklava (2 x 2 x 2-inch piece)	33	336
6 oz 1% milk	225	77

Total Calcium: 2,650 mg ○ **Total Calories: 2,028**

Basic Components

Calories 2,028	**Minerals**
Protein 124 g	Boron 8 mcg
Carbohydrates 200 g	Calcium 2,650 mg
Dietary Fiber 25 g	Copper 2 mg
Total Fat 84 g	Magnesium 330 mg
Saturated Fat 34 g	Manganese 2 mg
	Phosphorus 2,356 mg
Vitamins	Sodium 2,113 mg
Vitamin B6 2 mg	Zinc 12 mg
Vitamin B12 13 mcg	
Vitamin C 194 mg	
Vitamin D 487 IU	
Folate 420 mcg	
Vitamin K 36 mcg	

MENU FOR FRIDAY (DAY 12)

BREAKFAST	CALCIUM (mg)	CALORIES
3 egg-white omelette with	6	50
2 oz ricotta cheese	154	78
½ cup chopped celery	6	2
½ cup shredded carrot	3	5
½ cup sliced green peppers	1	4
2 Wasa® crackers	10	48
8 oz fortified orange juice	350	110

SNACK		
2 oz raisins	16	168
1 pear	18	98

LUNCH		
Tuna melt:		
3 oz tuna	12	109
1 oz low-fat, low-sodium cheddar		
melted on	199	49
1 slice whole-grain bread	24	65
1 cup spinach salad with	46	108
6 cherry tomatoes	5	21
2 tbsp oil and vinegar	9	139

SNACK		
2 plums	5	73
1 oz Brie	52	95

DINNER		
4 oz turkey breast (no skin) with	10	115
1 oz melted Swiss cheese	298	97
1 cup stewed okra	101	51
1 cup lima beans	26	115
1 cup sauteed kale	94	36
½ cup millet with chopped scallions and	21	112
1 tbsp chopped almonds	16	35

SNACK	CALCIUM	CALORIES
2 coconut macaroons	2	97
8 oz 1% milk	300	102

Total Calcium: 1,785 mg   ○   Total Calories: 1,981

Basic Components

Calories 1,981	Minerals
Protein 125 g	Boron 6 mcg
Carbohydrates 255 g	Calcium 1,785 mg
Dietary Fiber 32 g	Copper 2 mg
Total Fat 57 g	Magnesium 447 mg
Saturated Fat 23 g	Manganese 5 mg
	Phosphorus 1,744 mg
Vitamins	Sodium 1,560 mg
Vitamin B6 2 mg	Zinc 11 mg
Vitamin B12 4 mcg	
Vitamin C 258 mg	
Vitamin D 248 IU	
Folate 502 mcg	
Vitamin K 87 mcg	

MENU FOR SATURDAY (DAY 13)

BREAKFAST	CALCIUM (mg)	CALORIES
½ cup quick-cooking grits cooked with	1	145
1¼ cup low-fat milk topped with	450	165
2 tbsp cottage cheese	17	20
2 slices whole-grain toast	47	130
8 oz calcium-fortified Tropicana®		
grapefruit juice	400	90
Decaf coffee or tea		

SNACK		
1 kiwi	40	93
1 oz soy nuts	38	132

LUNCH		
1 cup macaroni and cheese (frozen variety)	280	319
1 cup tossed salad	46	26
2 tbsp oil and vinegar dressing	9	139
1 cup sauteed collard greens	226	49

SNACK		
1 nectarine	0	70

DINNER		
2 portobello mushrooms topped with	14	54
2 oz semisoft goat's milk cheese	169	206
1 oz roasted peppers	0	5
1 cup tossed salad	46	26
½ cup amaranth	75	182
1 cup steamed asparagus	36	43

SNACK	CALCIUM	CALORIES
¼ cup blackberries topped with	23	37
8 oz vanilla yogurt and a pinch of		
brown sugar	389	194

Total Calcium: 2,305 mg ○ **Total Calories: 2,126**

Basic Components

Calories 2,126	Minerals
Protein 99 g	Boron 2 mcg
Carbohydrates 309 g	Calcium 2,305 mg
Dietary Fiber 41 g	Copper 2 mg
Total Fat 65 g	Magnesium 401 mg
Saturated Fat 25 g	Manganese 6 mg
	Phosphorus 1,222 mg
Vitamins	Sodium 2,469 mg
Vitamin B6 2 mg	Zinc 9 mg
Vitamin B12 2 mcg	
Vitamin C 329 mg	
Vitamin D 159 IU	
Folate 890 mcg	
Vitamin K 7 mcg	

MENU FOR SUNDAY (DAY 14)

BREAKFAST	CALCIUM (mg)	CALORIES
2 whole-grain toaster waffles topped with	205	209
¼ cup low-fat vanilla yogurt	105	52
2 tbsp maple syrup	27	105
1 tbsp chopped almonds	16	35
1 cup low-fat milk	274	100
8 oz calcium-fortified Tropicana®		
orange juice	350	110

SNACK		
Wedge of honeydew melon		
with lemon juice	8	45

LUNCH		
3 oz grilled chicken in	12	168
1 whole-wheat pita bread with	10	170
½ cup chopped lettuce	10	4
½ sliced tomato	2	7
1 cup kale sauteed in garlic	94	36
1 cup steamed bok choy	158	20
½ cup couscous with	1	16
1 oz sauteed mushrooms	1	7

SNACK		
8 oz Tropicana® Strawberry Banana		
Smoothie	15	139
¼ cup hazelnuts	38	212

DINNER		
1 slice cheese pizza topped with		
broccoli and spinach	250	260
1 cup tossed salad	46	26
2 tbsp oil and vinegar	9	139

¾ cup raspberries	20	45
½ cup fat-free half and half	160	80

Total Calcium: 1,852 mg ○ **Total Calories: 2,000**

Basic Components

Calories 2,000	**Minerals**
Protein 90 g	Boron 3 mcg
Carbohydrates 270 g	Calcium 1,852 mg
Dietary Fiber 30 g	Copper 2 mg
Total Fat 69 g	Magnesium 318 mg
Saturated Fat 15 g	Manganese 8 mg
	Phosphorus 935 mg
Vitamins	Sodium 1,847 mg
Vitamin B6 2 mg	Zinc 8 mg
Vitamin B12 1 mcg	
Vitamin C 340 mg	
Vitamin D 155 IU	
Folate 485 mcg	
Vitamin K 122 mcg	

The 7-Day, Healthy, High-Calcium Diet for the Lactose-Intolerant

IF YOU ARE one of those people who have trouble digesting lactose (the sugar in milk) and dairy products, then this diet should work for you. As you know, there are enzymes you can take as a supplement to help you digest lactose, but this diet is lactose-free.

MENU FOR MONDAY (DAY 1)

BREAKFAST	CALCIUM (mg)	CALORIES
1 oz General Mills Total Raisin Bran®		
cereal	515	88
4 oz Silk® soy milk	139	46
1 whole-wheat English muffin	175	134
1 tbsp strawberry jam	0	50
Decaf coffee or tea		

SNACK		
1 Apple	0	80
Soy nuts	38	132

LUNCH		
4 oz hummus in	43	188
whole-wheat pita bread with	10	170
½ cup romaine lettuce	10	4
½ tomato	2	7
½ cup alfalfa sprouts	20	15
Decaf coffee or tea		

SNACK		
6 dried figs	164	291
¼ cup almonds	64	142

DINNER	CALCIUM	CALORIES
1 cup vegetarian baked beans		
sweetened with	127	236
1 tbsp blackstrap molasses	176	48
1 cup sauteed collard greens with garlic	226	49
½ cup brown rice	10	108
Decaf coffee or tea		

SNACK		
8 fl oz Lactaid® milk	505	95
2 coconut macaroons	2	97

Total Calcium: 2,225 mg ○ **Total Calories: 1,981**

Basic Components

Calories 1,981	**Minerals**
Protein 75 g	Boron 4 mcg
Carbohydrates 354 g	Calcium 2,225 mg
Dietary Fiber 63 g	Copper 3 mg
Total Fat 45 g	Magnesium 571 mg
Saturated Fat 9 g	Manganese 9 mg
	Phosphorus 1,406 mg
Vitamins	Sodium 2,631 mg
Vitamin B6 3 mg	Zinc 20 mg
Vitamin B12 5 mcg	
Vitamin C 68 mg	
Vitamin D 167 IU	
Folate 682 mcg	
Vitamin K 2 mcg	

MENU FOR TUESDAY (DAY 2)

BREAKFAST	CALCIUM (mg)	CALORIES
Tofu scramble:		
1 tsp olive oil	0	30
1 scallion	8	4
2 oz mushrooms	3	14
4 oz tofu	298	65
½ tomato	2	7
¼ green pepper	2	5
Pinch turmeric	1	1

Sauté scallion and mushrooms until tender, add remaining ingredients, and cool until heated through.

2 slices whole-grain toast	47	130
2 tsp margarine	0	67
8 oz calcium-fortified Tropicana®		
grapefruit juice	400	90
Decaf coffee or tea		

SNACK

2 kiwis	40	93
6 whole-wheat crackers	12	106

LUNCH

Salad:		
2 cups romaine lettuce	40	16
2 oz shredded carrots	13	22
2 oz green pepper	5	15
1 tomato	3	13
2 oz red cabbage	29	15
2 oz broccoli florets	27	16
½ cup chickpeas	40	134
½ cup black-eyed peas	21	100
Decaf coffee or tea		

SNACK	CALCIUM	CALORIES
1 oz almonds	77	171
6 oz Silk® apricot mango soy yogurt	500	160

DINNER		
4 oz grilled chicken breast	37	193
1 cup steamed bok choy	158	20
1 cup steamed snap green beans	58	44
½ cup brown rice	10	108
Decaf coffee or tea		

SNACK		
8 oz Lactaid® milk	550	103
2 oatmeal cookies	20	163

Total Calcium: 2,399 mg ○ **Total Calories: 1,904**

Basic Components

Calories 1,904	**Minerals**
Protein 89 g	Boron 9 mcg
Carbohydrates 287 g	Calcium 2,399 mg
Dietary Fiber 48 g	Copper 2 mg
Total Fat 56 g	Magnesium 515 mg
Saturated Fat 10 g	Manganese 6 mg
	Phosphorus 1,451 mg
Vitamins	Sodium 1,525 mg
Vitamin B6 2 mg	Zinc 9 mg
Vitamin B12 1 mcg	
Vitamin C 463 mg	
Vitamin D 142 IU	
Folate 827 mcg	
Vitamin K 68 mcg	

MENU FOR WEDNESDAY (DAY 3)

BREAKFAST	CALCIUM (mg)	CALORIES
2 Wasa® crackers with	10	48
2 tbsp almond butter	86	203
8 oz calcium-fortified Tropicana®		
orange juice	350	110
Decaf coffee or tea		

SNACK		
1 apple	0	80
¼ cup walnuts	25	164

LUNCH		
1 cup black beans in	46	227
2 corn tortillas topped with	91	115
½ cup lettuce	9	4
1 cup salsa	78	73
Decaf coffee or tea		

SNACK		
6 oz Silk® banana strawberry soy yogurt	500	160
1 peach	5	42

DINNER		
4 oz wild salmon	17	206
Mixed greens sauteed with garlic:		
½ cup collard greens	113	25
½ cup mustard greens	52	11
½ cup kale	47	18
½ cup chickpeas	40	134
½ cup amaranth	75	182
Decaf coffee or tea		

SNACK		
Smoothie:		
½ cup fortified orange juice	175	55

1 medium peach	5	42
1 small banana	5	75
½ cup blackberries	23	37
3 oz Silk® raspberry soy yogurt	250	80

Mix in blender until thoroughly combined.

Total Calcium: 2,001 mg   ◯   **Total Calories: 2,090**

Basic Components

Calories 2,090	Minerals
Protein 91 g	Boron 0 mcg
Carbohydrates 321 g	Calcium 2,001 mg
Dietary Fiber 61 g	Copper 4 mg
Total Fat 58 g	Magnesium 634 mg
Saturated Fat 7 g	Manganese 7 mg
	Phosphorus 1,530 mg
Vitamins	Sodium 1,436 mg
Vitamin B6 3 mg	Zinc 10 mg
Vitamin B12 3 mcg	
Vitamin C 307 mg	
Vitamin D 318 IU	
Folate 906 mcg	
Vitamin K 40 mcg	

MENU FOR THURSDAY (DAY 4)

BREAKFAST	CALCIUM (mg)	CALORIES
Smoothie:		
¼ cup Silk® soy milk	75	25
6 oz Silk® strawberry soy yogurt	500	160
2 tbsp calcium-fortified orange juice	44	14
1 tbsp blackstrap molasses	176	48
½ cup blueberries	4	41
½ cup strawberries	11	23
1 small banana	5	75
Decaf coffee or tea		

SNACK		
1 toaster corn muffin	6	114
2 tsp margarine	0	67

LUNCH		
1 falafel patty 2.25" diameter with	9	57
¼ cup tahini	79	340
½ cup lettuce	9	4
1 tomato	3	13
1 cup stewed okra in tomato sauce	112	75
Decaf coffee or tea		

SNACK		
2 x 2 x 2.5–1 inch piece baklava	33	336
8 oz Silk® soy milk	300	100

DINNER		
4 oz broiled fillet of sole	20	133
½ cup roasted, steamed buckwheat with	6	77
1 oz mushrooms	1	7
1 cup sauteed collard greens	226	49
Decaf coffee or tea		

SNACK	CALCIUM	CALORIES
8 oz Lactaid® milk	550	103
4 graham crackers	7	120

Total Calcium: 2,177 mg ○ **Total Calories: 1,980**

Basic Components

Calories 1,980	**Minerals**
Protein 84 g	Boron 6 mcg
Carbohydrates 236 g	Calcium 2,177 mg
Dietary Fiber 30 g	Copper 2 mg
Total Fat 85 g	Magnesium 618 mg
Saturated Fat 19 g	Manganese 5 mg
	Phosphorus 1,507 mg
Vitamins	Sodium 1,411 mg
Vitamin B6 2 mg	Zinc 12 mg
Vitamin B12 8 mcg	
Vitamin C 166 mg	
Vitamin D 345 IU	
Folate 506 mcg	
Vitamin K 39 mcg	

MENU FOR FRIDAY (DAY 5)

BREAKFAST	CALCIUM (mg)	CALORIES
Soy yogurt parfait:		
6 oz Silk® vanilla soy yogurt	500	120
1 oz granola cereal	34	145
½ cup blackberries	23	37
Decaf coffee or tea		

SNACK		
2 Wasa® crackers	10	48
2 tbsp cashew butter	14	188

LUNCH		
Sardine pasta salad:		
4 oz whole-wheat pasta elbows	17	141
1 3-oz can sardines	351	191
¼ cup chopped parsley	21	5
1 tbsp lemon juice	1	4
1 tbsp olive oil	0	119
2 tbsp chopped scallion	0	5
1 cup tossed salad	46	26
2 Wasa® crackers	10	48
Decaf coffee or tea		

SNACK		
1 cup grapes	13	62
¼ cup almonds	64	142

DINNER		
Grilled tofu sandwich:		
4 oz grilled tofu	397	86
2 slices whole-grain toast	47	130
8 oz fat-free five-bean		
vegetable soup (canned)	76	132
1 cup tossed salad	46	26

4 oz peas and pearl onions   26   79
Decaf coffee or tea

SNACK

½ cup Rice Dream® vanilla Swiss almond
    frozen dessert   25   222

Total Calcium: 1,721 mg ○ **Total Calories: 1,955**

Basic Components

Calories	1,955	Minerals	
Protein 84 g		Boron 2 mcg	
Carbohydrates 237 g		Calcium 1,721 mg	
Dietary Fiber 43 g		Copper 2 mg	
Total Fat 84 g		Magnesium 398 mg	
Saturated Fat 13 g		Manganese 7 mg	
		Phosphorus 1,252 mg	
Vitamins		Sodium 1,393 mg	
Vitamin B6 1 mg		Zinc 8 mg	
Vitamin B12 8 mcg			
Vitamin C 125 mg			
Vitamin D 250 IU			
Folate 416 mcg			
Vitamin K 88 mcg			

MENU FOR SATURDAY (DAY 6)

BREAKFAST	CALCIUM (mg)	CALORIES
8 oz café latte (4 oz decaf coffee +		
4 oz hot Lactaid® milk)	253	47
1 low-fat oat bran muffin	30	160
Decaf coffee or tea		

SNACK		
2 oz trail mix	44	262
1 Granny Smith apple	7	61

LUNCH		
Tuna sandwich:		
1 6-oz can tuna in water	24	220
1 tbsp light mayonnaise	1	50
½ cup shredded lettuce	9	4
1 tomato	3	13
2 slices whole-wheat bread	47	130
1 cup spinach salad	46	108
2 tbsp low-cal Italian dressing	0	29
Decaf coffee or tea		

SNACK		
6 oz Silk® vanilla soy yogurt covered with	500	120
½ cup strawberries and	12	25
½ cup blackberries	23	37

DINNER		
4 oz perch breaded with	155	137
¼ cup crushed fortified Total® cereal	188	21
Basmati rice with shallots, white beans,		
and watercress:		
1 tbsp shallots, *sauteed in*	4	7
1 tsp olive oil, *add*	0	40

½ cup basmati rice, *sauté, and*	2	57
add 1 cup water		
Simmer until rice is tender, add		
¼ cup white beans,	33	64
1 cup chopped watercress *and*		
heat through	41	4
1 cup sauteed kale	94	36
Decaf coffee or tea		

SNACK

8 oz Lactaid® milk	550	103
4 oz Mrs. Smith's® apple cobbler	0	252

Total Calcium: 2,066 mg ○ **Total Calories: 1,990**

Basic Components

Calories 1,990	Minerals
Protein 118 g	Boron 6 mcg
Carbohydrates 248 g	Calcium 2,066 mg
Dietary Fiber 29 g	Copper 1 mg
Total Fat 64 g	Magnesium 404 mg
Saturated Fat 14 g	Manganese 4 mg
	Phosphorus 1,725 mg
Vitamins	Sodium 2,469 mg
Vitamin B6 2 mg	Zinc 10 mg
Vitamin B12 6 mcg	
Vitamin C 175 mg	
Vitamin D 471 IU	
Folate 404 mcg	
Vitamin K 126 mcg	

MENU FOR SUNDAY (DAY 7)

BREAKFAST	CALCIUM (mg)	CALORIES
1 packet fortified instant oatmeal		
cooked in	161	103
6 oz almond milk	144	44
2 tbsp raisins	5	54
1 whole-wheat English muffin	175	134
2 tsp margarine	0	67
Decaf coffee or tea		

SNACK		
2 celery sticks with	40	20
1 tbsp peanut butter	9	93

LUNCH		
4 oz turkey breast	24	214
2 pieces Hollywood Dark®		
high-calcium bread	274	77
1 tsp fat free mayonnaise	0	4
1 tsp Dijon mustard	0	5
½ cup lettuce	9	4
1 tomato	3	13
1 cup tossed green salad	46	26
2 tbsp oil and vinegar	9	139
Decaf coffee or tea		

SNACK		
6 oz Silk® peach soy yogurt	500	170
1 medium peach	5	42

DINNER		
Chinese stir-fry:		
3 oz stir-fried tofu	817	230
½ cup stir-fried bok choy	79	10
½ cup stir-fried broccoli	17	10

½ cup stir-fried carrots	24	35
½ cup stir-fried Chinese cabbage	89	11
½ cup stir-fried snow peas	34	34
½ cup fried rice with bean sprouts and scallions	14	135
Decaf coffee or tea		

SNACK

½ cup Rice Dream® cocoa fudge frozen dessert with	20	150
2 tbsp chocolate syrup	6	102
2 tbsp shredded coconut	2	58

Total Calcium: 2,507 mg ○ **Total Calories: 1,985**

Basic Components

Calories 1,985	Minerals
Protein 86 g	Boron 2 mcg
Carbohydrates 245 g	Calcium 2,507 mg
Dietary Fiber 34 g	Copper 1 mg
Total Fat 81 g	Magnesium 385 mg
Saturated Fat 15 g	Manganese 6 mg
	Phosphorus 1,270 mg
Vitamins	Sodium 1,895 mg
Vitamin B6 3 mg	Zinc 9 mg
Vitamin B12 0 mcg	
Vitamin C 156 mg	
Vitamin D 84 IU	
Folate 459 mcg	
Vitamin K 62 mcg	

The 7-Day, Healthy, High-Calcium Diet for Vegetarians

MOST OF THE VEGETARIANS I know are careful to eat a balanced diet every day. If you are a vegetarian and have no trouble digesting the lactose in milk, then this diet should work well for you. Notice that I've included a few recipe suggestions in this diet, but feel free to substitute other simple-to-prepare foods if you'd like.

MENU FOR MONDAY (DAY 1)

BREAKFAST	CALCIUM (mg)	CALORIES
8 oz Tropicana® calcium-fortified grapefruit juice	400	90
1 cup Total® cereal	1,000	110
1 cup skim or 1% or 2% milk	300	102
1 whole grain English muffin	175	134
1 tbsp jam	4	48

LUNCH		
1 bowl vegetarian split-pea soup	40	110
Vegetable pasta salad, sprinkled with	96	383
2 tbsp grated Parmesan cheese	138	46
2 oz oat bran pita bread	10	170
1 oz Edam cheese	207	101

DINNER		
6 oz veggie burger on whole-grain bun with lettuce, tomato, and low-fat mayonnaise	248	442
Green beans with slivered almonds	54	60

Cucumber and tomato salad topped
    with 1 oz cheddar cheese   214   134
Strawberry yogurt surprise* (½ recipe)   335   220

*Indicates that there is a recipe in the Cookbook section.

Total Calcium: 3,228 mg   ○   Total Calories: 2,258

Basic Components

Calories 2,258	Minerals
Protein 105.51 g	Boron 6.57 mcg
Carbohydrates 359.07 g	Calcium 3,228 mg
Dietary Fiber 43.08 g	Copper 1.38 mg
Total Fat 59.21 g	Magnesium 439.49 mg
Saturated Fat 25.51 g	Manganese 4.78 mg
	Phosphorus 2,128.62 mg
Vitamins	Sodium 3,977.27 mg
Vitamin B6 4.22 mg	Zinc 19.02 mg
Vitamin B12 7.07 mcg	
Vitamin C 300.99 mg	
Vitamin D 214.17 IU	
Folate 558.33 mcg	
Vitamin K 52.1 mcg	

MENU FOR TUESDAY (DAY 2)

BREAKFAST	CALCIUM (mg)	CALORIES
1 cup plain, low-fat yogurt topped with	415	143
2 tbsp honey	3	129
2 slices calcium-fortified whole-		
grain bread	277	78
2 tbsp jam	8	99
1 California navel orange	56	64

LUNCH		
Grilled cheddar cheese, tomato, and onion		
sandwich on whole-grain bread	651	295
Healthy greens with sun-dried tomato		
salad, oil and vinegar dressing	51	176
topped with		
1 oz grated Swiss cheese	272	106

DINNER		
Cream of asparagus soup (canned,		
made with low-fat milk)	159	147
11 oz vegetable lasagne	291	392
1 cup Caesar salad	40	113
4 oz frozen low-fat vanilla yogurt	180	119
topped with		
2 tbsp chocolate syrup and		
chopped pecans	17	204

Total Calcium: 2,420 mg ○ **Total Calories: 2,065**

Basic Components

Calories 2,065	Minerals
Protein 82.66 g	Boron 2.09 mcg
Carbohydrates 245.89 g	Calcium 2,420 mg
Dietary Fiber 22.69 g	Copper 1.25 mg
Total Fat 88.25 g	Magnesium 284.23 mg
Saturated Fat 30.86 g	Manganese 3.04 mg
	Phosphorus 1,753 mg
Vitamins	Sodium 3,162.62 mg
Vitamin B6 1.13 mg	Zinc 11.69 mg
Vitamin B12 3.7 mcg	
Vitamin C 205.77 mg	
Vitamin D 17.88 IU	
Vitamin K 4.69 mcg	

MENU FOR WEDNESDAY (DAY 3)

BREAKFAST	CALCIUM (mg)	CALORIES
8 oz glass Tropicana®		
calcium-fortified orange juice	350	90
1 waffle with 3 tbsp	77	88
maple syrup	40	157
½ cup sliced strawberries	11	23

LUNCH		
Veggie melt Chopped fresh vegetables on		
toasted English muffin topped with	175	134
2 slices of Swiss cheese	800	260
Put under broiler until cheese		
has melted.		
Arugula and endive salad with		
blue cheese dressing	25	160

DINNER		
Fettuccine with four cheeses		
(1 oz each)	960	922
Broccoli with lemon and 2 tbsp sliced		
almonds	66	91
Garlic bread	0	160
Butterscotch pudding*	163	161

Total Calcium: 2,667 mg　○　**Total Calories: 2,246**

Basic Components

Calories 2,246		**Minerals**	
Protein 90.02 g		Boron 2.05 mcg	
Carbohydrates 229.75 g		Calcium 2,667 mg	
Dietary Fiber 17.52 g		Copper 0.77 mg	
Total Fat 119.76 g		Magnesium 244 mg	
Saturated Fat 59.38 g		Manganese 4.04 mg	
		Phosphorus	
Vitamins		1,767.92 mg	
Vitamin B6 1.06 mg		Sodium 2,454.94 mg	
Vitamin B12 2.42 mcg		Zinc 12.02 mg	
Vitamin C 266.57 mg			
Vitamin D 125.78 IU			
Folate 435.75 mcg			
Vitamin K 87.86 mcg			

MENU FOR THURSDAY (DAY 4)

BREAKFAST	CALCIUM (mg)	CALORIES
8 oz glass Tropicana®		
calcium-fortified orange juice	350	110
2 6-inch banana pancakes with	194	299
3 tbsp maple syrup	40	157

LUNCH		
Avocado, tomato, onion, and shredded		
Swiss cheese sandwich on		
whole-grain pita bread or toast	825	511
½ cup potato salad made with low-fat		
mayonnaise	15	106
6 Pepperidge Farm® cheese sticks	27	93

DINNER		
Steamed vegetable plate (1 cup broccoli,		
cauliflower, spinach)	75	37
Watercress and arugula salad with 2 oz.		
grated Parmesan cheese	153	49
Cheese grits*	527	439
Frozen yogurt parfait topped with fresh		
strawberries, blueberries, and		
raspberries	187	144

Total Calcium: 2,393 mg ○ **Total Calories: 1,945**

Basic Components

Calories	1,945		Minerals	
Protein	58.82 g		Boron	0.55 mcg
Carbohydrates	231.79 g		Calcium	2,393 mg
Dietary Fiber	20.25 g		Copper	0.59 mg
Total Fat	42.43 g		Magnesium	170.1 mg
Saturated Fat	19.03 g		Manganese	4.59 mg
			Phosphorus	
Vitamins				1,454.71 mg
Vitamin B6	0.94 mg		Sodium	2,642.69 mg
Vitamin B12	1 mcg		Zinc	9.04 mg
Vitamin C	228.11 mg			
Vitamin D	80.88 IU			
Folate	253.23 mcg			
Vitamin K	44.95 mcg			

MENU FOR FRIDAY (DAY 5)

BREAKFAST	CALCIUM (mg)	CALORIES
8 oz glass Tropicana®		
grapefruit juice	400	90
2 eggs scrambled with sauteed onions		
and 1 tbsp powdered milk	115	173
1 slice whole-grain toast	24	65

LUNCH		
Eggplant parmigiana	420	366
Tomato, avocado, and cucumber salad		
with poppy-seed dressing	31	331
Whole-grain roll	38	96

DINNER		
Cheese soup (canned, made with		
low-fat milk)	261	209
1 cup spaghetti with broccoli rabe	35	177
whole-grain French bread with garlic		
butter	7	216
2 whole-grain crackers with 1 oz		
cheese	416	307

Total Calcium: 1,747 mg ○ **Total Calories: 2,030**

Basic Components

Calories 2,030		**Minerals**	
Protein 86.05 g		Boron 2.59 mcg	
Carbohydrates 212.22 g		Calcium 1,747 mg	
Dietary Fiber 19.91 g		Copper 1.16 mg	
Total Fat 124.8 g		Magnesium 254.24 mg	
Saturated Fat 49.82 g		Manganese 2.49 mg	
		Phosphorus	
Vitamins		1,559.43 mg	
Vitamin B6 1.18 mg		Sodium 4,281.52 mg	
Vitamin B12 3.34 mcg		Zinc 9.48 mg	
Vitamin C 167.2 mg			
Vitamin D 121.3 IU			
Folate 360.77 mcg			
Vitamin K 24.31 mcg			

MENU FOR SATURDAY (DAY 6)

BREAKFAST	CALCIUM (mg)	CALORIES
1 cup low-fat yogurt with		
2 tbsp honey and	250	240
chopped pecans	8	180
1 whole-grain English muffin,		
topped with 1 oz melted		
cheddar cheese	584	363
1 orange	56	64

LUNCH		
Cheese and broccoli/cauliflower		
casserole	320	236
Arugula salad with shaved Parmesan	101	28
Fruit salad topped with low-fat sour cream	63	148

DINNER		
Spaghetti primavera with 3 tbsp		
grated Parmesan	306	308
Watercress and 1 oz baked goat cheese		
salad, sprinkled with 1 oz chopped		
walnuts	557	276
Whole-grain French bread	71	262
Mixed-melon fruit salad	19	62

Total Calcium: 2,335 mg ○ **Total Calories: 2,167**

Basic Components

Calories	2,167	Minerals	
Protein	94.64 g	Boron	1.05 mcg
Carbohydrates	260.78 g	Calcium	2,335 mg
Dietary Fiber	20.16 g	Copper	1.3 mg
Total Fat	90.03 g	Magnesium	255.31 mg
Saturated Fat	46.14 g	Manganese	3.96 mg
		Phosphorus	
Vitamins			1,583.22 mg
Vitamin B6	0.97 mg	Sodium	2,885.98 mg
Vitamin B12	1.4 mcg	Zinc	8.07 mg
Vitamin C	140.7 mg		
Vitamin D	59.99 IU		
Folate	240.18 mcg		
Vitamin K	92.84 mcg		

MENU FOR SUNDAY (DAY 7)

BREAKFAST	CALCIUM (mg)	CALORIES
1 half grapefruit	20	60
1 two-egg cheese omelette	594	362
1 slice whole-grain toast with jam	32	162

LUNCH		
1½ cups green pea soup (canned, made with low-fat milk)	419	579
One sliced tomato and 2 oz mozzarella salad	296	172
Open-face grilled cheddar cheese and onion sandwich	435	299

DINNER		
Cheese soufflé	218	226
Endive, watercress, and arugula salad with blue cheese vinaigrette dressing	74	163
Baked, breaded tomatoes (topped with bread crumbs, grated Parmesan cheese, and parsley)	210	183
Sliced strawberries topped with low-fat sour cream and brown sugar	98	120

Total Calcium: 2,396 mg ○ **Total Calories: 2,326**

Basic Components

Calories	2,326	Minerals	
Protein 120.53 g		Boron 4.55 mcg	
Carbohydrates 217.42 g		Calcium 2,396 mg	
Dietary Fiber 25.9 g		Copper 1.51 mg	
Total Fat 120.49 g		Magnesium 305.48 mg	
Saturated Fat 61.19 g		Manganese 3.69 mg	
		Phosphorus 2,221.97 mg	
Vitamins		Sodium 5,251.01 mg	
Vitamin B6 1.14 mg		Zinc 13.75 mg	
Vitamin B12 4.94 mcg			
Vitamin C 208.52 mg			
Vitamin D 263.49 IU			
Folate 288.01 mcg			
Vitamin K 114.64 mcg			

CHAPTER TEN

THE SIMPLE, LONG-TERM EATING PROGRAM TO MAXIMIZE BONE STRENGTH

Thirty Tips on How to Add Calcium to Your Everyday Diet

L ET FOOD BE YOUR MEDICINE, and medicine be your food." You know who said that? It was Hippocrates, the father of modern medicine, in 500 B.C. He may not have had the benefit of all our sophisticated, scientific research into the nutritional values of various foods, but he knew one thing that is as true today as it was 2,500 years ago: If you eat a variety of fresh (or slightly processed) foods, with an emphasis on fruits, vegetables, and whole grains and a modest amount of meats and fish thrown in, you'll be getting all the nutrition you need to stay healthy, active, and disease-free.

The modern-day science of nutrition has become highly complex, and even some of the best nutritionists I know sometimes get a little confused by all the conflicting statistics on just how much of what you should eat each day. For our purposes, though, we are going to simplify the complex science of nutrition by concentrating on how to get the maximum amount of calcium into your daily diet, while making sure you get what most nutritionists agree are healthy amounts of all the other important nutrients.

Before I get into the calcium discussion, I want to mention one of the amazing new findings to come out of all this research into foods and how they nourish us. Recently, scientists have discovered substances in foods—especially plant foods—that are not vitamins and not minerals, but are essential to good health. These substances are called *phytochemicals*. There are about four thousand of them (though only 150 of them have been carefully studied) and they provide the color-giving pigments in plants. Like a painter's palette, they are responsible for

> ### Put a Rainbow on Your Plate
>
> Try to eat a variety of brightly colored foods each day to take advantage of the health-giving *phytochemicals* that give them their color. Eat at least one food from the **red group**, the **green group**, the **yellow-orange group**, and the **purple-blue group**.

making bananas yellow, tomatoes red, blueberries blue, and broccoli green. That's not all, though. Some of these brightly colored vegetables seem to interfere with the synthesis of cholesterol in the body, and so may help protect our arteries. There are others that act as antioxidants, meaning they reduce the damaging effects of free radicals and thereby help protect us against diabetes, cancer, and other serious diseases. Research from the Tufts University USDA Human Nutrition Research Center on Aging suggests that eating brightly colored foods can significantly increase the antioxidant power in our bloodstream. The ORAC (oxygen radical absorbance capacity) scores for 3.5 ounces of some of the colorful foods that are particularly high in these antioxidants, according to the Tufts researchers are:

FRUITS

- Prunes (5,770)
- Raisins (2,830)
- Blueberries (2,400)
- Strawberries (1,504)
- Raspberries (1,220)
- Plums (949)
- Oranges (750)
- Red grapes (739)

VEGETABLES

- Kale (1,770)

- Spinach (1,260)

- Brussels sprouts (980)

- Broccoli florets (890)

- Beets (840)

- Red bell peppers (710)

- Yellow corn (400)

- Eggplant (390)

- Carrots (210)

Whole books have been written about the importance of keeping colorful foods in your diet. Now that we have all this new information about the importance of phytochemicals, I must say that I have become a convert. When you think food, think color. Colorful foods are not only pleasing to the eye, they also lower cholesterol and are storehouses of healthy antioxidants.

Now, back to calcium. You already know what the best food sources of calcium are: low-fat milk, cheese and dairy products, low-fat yogurt, green leafy vegetables, canned sardines and salmon, nuts, legumes, tofu processed with calcium carbonate, and whole grains. Calcium-fortified foods like cereal, breads, and juices are good calcium sources, too, so I'd suggest you buy those whenever you can.

You can make things easier on yourself, and ensure that you'll have enough high-calcium food in your cupboard, if you simply stock up on these simple items every week when you do your grocery shopping. This is a bare-bones list (I thought that phrase was appropriate) and there are a lot of other calcium-rich foods for you to choose from when you do your shopping. But if you make sure you have these items in your house, you won't run short on foods rich in natural calcium.

My Bare-Bones Weekly Grocery List

1. Calcium-fortified Tropicana® grapefruit juice
2. Calcium-fortified Tropicana® orange juice with vitamin D
3. Skim or low-fat milk
4. 1-cup containers of plain, low-fat yogurt
5. Parmesan cheese
6. Cheddar cheese
7. Calcium-fortified cereal such as Total® or Product 19®
8. Canned sardines with bones, and salmon with bones

Once you have all these foods at home, then follow my simple, three-step everyday to-do list and you'll be in business.

My Three-Step, Everyday To-Do List

1. Drink an eight-ounce glass of calcium-fortified orange juice or grapefruit juice, or low-fat 1% milk, every morning at breakfast. This will give you 300 mg of calcium right off the bat.
2. Eat one cup of plain, low-fat yogurt each day, either at breakfast, as a snack, or before you go to bed. Add a little fresh fruit and some chopped nuts if you'd like. This will give you at least another 450 mg of calcium.
3. Take one ounce of hard Parmesan or cheddar cheese and grate it over your vegetables, potato, salad, or even fish at dinner. Count on this for another 330 mg of calcium or so.

That's it. If you stock up on these groceries and follow these three simple little steps every day, you will automatically be getting between 1,000 and 1,200 mg of calcium in your daily diet with very little effort at all. When you consider that more than half of all Americans eat less than 600 mg of calcium a day, you can see how far ahead of the game you'll be.

Here are some other easy and delicious ways to get more calcium into your daily diet.

THIRTY WAYS TO LOVE YOUR BEAUTIFUL BONES

Tips on How to Add
Calcium to Your Everyday Diet

1. Sprinkle an ounce of shredded Parmesan or cheddar cheese on baked potatoes, soups, salads, green vegetables (all vegetables for that matter), and casseroles. Okay, I mentioned this before, but because it is such a tasty and simple way to get more calcium into your diet, I wanted to mention it again. You can add roughly 330 mg of calcium to your diet by shredding one ounce of hard Parmesan cheese.

2. Make your oatmeal and hot chocolate with skim milk instead of water. You might toss in some nonfat dry milk to really up the calcium.

3. Instead of coffee, try a latte, which is half coffee (preferably decaf) and half hot skim milk.

4. Drink an eight-ounce glass of calcium-fortified orange juice or calcium-fortified grapefruit juice every day. That's 350 mg of calcium right there.

5. Melt low-fat cheddar or Swiss cheese on your calcium-fortified toast or bagel at breakfast in the morning.

6. Try a plain, low-fat yogurt with a tablespoon of honey on it as a mid-afternoon snack.

7. Drink the rest of the milk in the bowl after you've finished your dry cereal.

8. Add two or three tablespoons of nonfat dry milk to cream soups, creamy salad dressings, casseroles, and smoothies. This could give you a whopping 400 extra mg of calcium.

9. Drink a glass of skim or low-fat milk at night before you go to bed. It may sound like kid's stuff, but it's great for your bones. Add a little chocolate syrup and heat it up if you really want a treat.

10. Substitute plain, low-fat yogurt for some of the mayonnaise in salad dressings, dips, and on sandwiches.

11. Add a little low-fat milk and sour cream to goat cheese to make a

delicious dip for raw vegetables and vegetable chips. You might want to toss in a few chopped onions, too.

12. At lunch, for a change, try canned salmon or sardines with lettuce, tomato, and onions, instead of tuna.

13. Use calcium-fortified bread or toast for your sandwiches. It is not always easy to find, so you might have to check with a health-food store and ask them to order it for you.

14. Have fruit and cheese with crackers for dessert a couple of times a week.

15. Make a tuna melt or salmon melt by putting some tuna or salmon salad on a toasted English muffin, topping it with two slices of Swiss cheese, and running it under the broiler for a couple of minutes.

16. Top fresh strawberries, blueberries, or fruit salad with a big dollop of low-fat sour cream and a pinch of brown sugar.

17. Add a slice or two of cheese to your sandwich at lunch when appropriate. Obviously, this won't work with peanut butter and jelly.

18. Whenever a recipe calls for orange juice, use fortified orange juice instead of regular.

19. Mix a cup of plain low-fat yogurt, two to three tablespoons granola, and a little fresh fruit for a pick-me-up in the afternoon.

20. Substitute skim milk, or low-fat 1% milk, for water when cooking pancakes, waffles, biscuits, and grits.

21. Add two tablespoons blackstrap molasses to your syrup the next time you have pancakes or waffles.

22. Use a teaspoon or two of nonfat powdered dry milk in your coffee or tea instead of whole or low-fat milk. Try to switch to decaffeinated coffee if you can. Personally, I cannot taste the difference.

23. Add three tablespoons grated Parmesan cheese to your microwave popcorn. Season with a little celery salt. Delicious!

24. Mix four ounces calcium-fortified orange juice with four ounces calcium-fortified grapefruit juice and drink as a pick-me-up during the day. Try this or simply an eight-ounce glass of calcium-fortified grapefruit juice as a cocktail before dinner if you are trying to lose weight.

25. Make a sardine spread for crackers by mixing one six-ounce can of mashed sardines with the juice of half a lemon and three tablespoons

sour cream. Keep it covered in the refrigerator in a glass bowl until ready to use.

26. **Make a dip for raw vegetables by mixing one cup ricotta cheese with half a package of dried onion soup mix.** Taste it and add more of the soup mix if you'd like.
27. **Whenever possible, buy calcium-fortified juices, breads, and cereals.**
28. **Enjoy frozen yogurt topped with fresh berries, or sliced bananas with chopped nuts for dessert.**
29. **Mix an eight-ounce can of salmon with chopped celery, serve on a bed of watercress topped with light mayonnaise or your favorite salad dressing for a delightful, low-calorie lunch.**
30. **Mix up a large batch of your favorite smoothie in the morning (see page 170) and drink a five- to eight-ounce glass as a snack a couple of times a day.**

WHAT DOES THIS HAVE TO DO WITH ME?

Just everything, that's all. If you conscientiously set out to change your lifestyle by making sure you get 1,500 mg of calcium in your diet every day, and by taking up a gentle exercise program (which we'll talk about in Chapter 11), then you'll be taking a giant step toward protecting yourself from the pain and powerlessness often caused by osteoporosis. Not only that, I predict that in a matter of weeks you'll start to feel better than you have in a long time.

PART THREE

BUILD BETTER BONES WITH EXERCISE

BONES NEED EXERCISE LIKE BABIES NEED LOVE

The Simple Weight-Bearing, Muscle-Building Workout Program That Guarantees Results

ABIES NEED TO BE LOVED, touched, nourished, and nurtured to develop into healthy children and adults. We all know that. So it is with our bones, too. Providing a well-balanced, high-calcium diet goes a long way toward keeping our bones in tip-top shape, but a healthy diet can't do the job alone. Our bones *need* exercise, as do our bodies, for that matter. If a healthy person on a high-calcium diet is confined to bed rest for an extended period of time, that person will develop osteopenia, the precursor of osteoporosis, in which the bones become less dense and more brittle. Exercise is essential. Bones respond to stress. In fact, if they are not sufficiently stressed, they begin to weaken, as I've just indicated. Use it or lose it, as they say.

There are two basic types of exercises to strengthen bones. One is weight-bearing activities like walking or running, which constantly put stress on the bones. The other is building up muscle. The muscles that are attached to our bones move our joints and stimulate bone production and growth. For most normal people, the daily activities of walking, carrying, lifting, and bending go a long way toward keeping our bones healthy. However, if you are over fifty, have a predisposition toward osteoporosis, or have suffered an extended illness, these routine activities will not be enough.

I have learned the hard way that if I give my patients a complicated exercise program, their enthusiasm and dedication dwindle quickly. Therefore, my exercise menu is simple and easily accomplished, and you don't have to go to a gym or invest in special equipment. All you need is what you already have, and the wisdom and determination to make my exercises an integral part of your life. I have developed one series of exercises for people who are generally healthy and don't have to restrict their activities because of special conditions such as heart trouble, rheumatoid arthritis, respiratory difficulties, or advanced osteoporosis.

These programs only require fifteen to twenty minutes a day, and consist of weight-bearing, muscle-strengthening, and stretching exercises. In addition to my exercise regimen, I have also developed a ten-point system to help my patients work in a little exercise while they are going about their daily lives. I encourage them to use it throughout each day. And remember, this is to be done in addition to—not instead of—my regular exercise routine. Here's how it works.

THE TEN-POINT SYSTEM

Just as eating lots of absorbable calcium at just one meal a day will not give your body all the calcium it needs, exercising just once a day won't do the whole job, either. There are many simple tasks you can perform all day long, and once you have earned your "ten points" you can feel confident that you have done enough exercise on that day to keep your bones happy. You don't have to get ten points every single day. If, for example, you get twelve points one day, you can carry them over to the next day, when you'll try to get eight points, and vice versa. Carrying points over for one day is fine, but not for two days. The whole point of the point system is to keep yourself moving, and even though it may seem difficult at first, don't get discouraged. Just remember that you are doing one of the best things possible for yourself, so get up and get a move on. Here's how the Ten-Point System works:

Walking up two flights of stairs	1 point
Walking ten blocks at a brisk pace	2 points
Carrying groceries	½ point
Working in the garden for an hour	2 points
Cleaning out your closet	1 point
Dancing for fifteen minutes	1 point
Taking a two-mile bike ride	2 points
Playing eighteen holes of golf with a cart	2 points

Playing one set of singles tennis	4 points
Playing one set of doubles tennis	3 points
Shoveling snow for fifteen minutes	1 point
Shooting baskets with your kids or grandkids	1 point
Running around a city block	2 points
Carrying packages to the post office	1 point
Swimming thirty laps	6 points
Water aerobics for one hour	8 points
Brisk walking for thirty minutes	8 points
Jogging for thirty minutes	8 points
Bicycling for thirty minutes	8 points
Working out at the gym for forty-five minutes	10 points

If you have followed the Fifteen-Minute Morning Exercise Routine that I'm about to explain, then you'll have the whole rest of the day to earn your ten points. Concentrate on changing your habits in little ways at first. You might take the stairs to your office if you work on a low floor, or carry your groceries to the car yourself instead of having someone at the store do it for you. If you are visiting a neighbor a few blocks away, walk, don't drive. Take every opportunity you can to get your body out and about. It won't be long before you'll start to feel the difference.

THE FIFTEEN-MINUTE MORNING EXERCISE ROUTINE

Most of my patients prefer to do these simple exercises as soon as they get out of bed. That way they have done something good for themselves before they even take their morning shower and start to get ready for the day ahead.

GROUP A

Stretching and Breathing

Always start with simple stretching. This is especially important if you've just gotten out of bed. Every exercise program that can trace its origins to

Eastern philosophy, from Yoga to tai chi, stresses relaxation and deep breathing, and so does my exercise program. These exercises should be done slowly.

❶ Deep Breathing (thirty seconds)

Stand erect, shoulders back, stomach in, head high, hands at your side. Slowly lift your hands away from the side of your body with your elbows straight, until they are well above the level of your shoulders. As you do this, gradually take a deep breath through your mouth and fill your lungs with air. Hold your breath for ten seconds. Bring your arms down as slowly as you raised them while exhaling completely. Repeat three times.

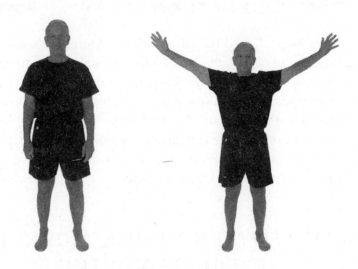

❷ Calf-Muscle Stretch (one minute)

Stand facing the wall. Put your right foot about two foot lengths behind the left. Place the palms of your hands against the wall, lean forward, keeping your back straight and head up. Bend your left knee but keep your right foot flat on the floor, heel down. As you bend the left knee also bend your elbows and bring your body toward the wall. You should feel a pulling sensation in your right calf muscle. Hold for ten seconds. It is very important to properly stretch the muscle. Repeat three times on the right, then reverse feet and do the same exercise with the left foot back. Remember, it is the calf muscle in the back leg that is getting the stretch.

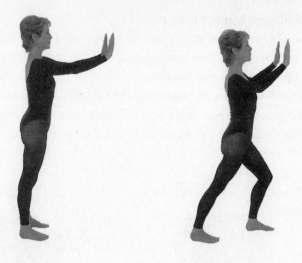

③ The Hamstring Stretch (one minute)

Place your leftt foot on a low chair. Turn your right foot to the side. The heel of your left foot should rest on top of the chair with the toes pointed toward the ceiling. Place your left hand on your left thigh. Slowly bend the right knee keeping your back straight until you feel a pull in the muscle behind your left thigh and knee (the hamstring muscles). Hold for ten seconds. Repeat three times. Switch and do the same exercise with the opposite leg.

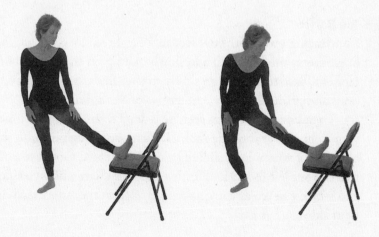

④ The Adductor Stretch (one minute)

Stand with your feet wide apart and your hands on your waist. Turn your left foot away from your body. Bend your left knee, keeping your right knee straight until you feel a pull in your right groin (keeping your left knee bent). You are stretching the left adductor muscles. Hold for ten seconds and repeat three times. Repeat the exercise with your right foot out. Bend your right knee and stretch your right adductor muscles.

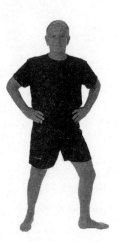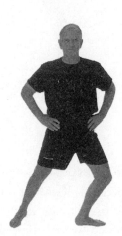

Strengthening

① Toe Raises

Stand facing a wall with your feet about eighteen inches apart. Put your fingertips against the wall and slowly rise up on the toes of both feet. Hold for five seconds. Drop slowly to your heels. Start with five repetitions and gradually increase to ten as you get stronger.

The second part of this exercise is done with one leg at a time. Keep your fingertips against the wall. Lift your right thigh up with the knee bent. All of your weight should be on the left foot. Slowly rise onto the toes of your left foot. Hold for five seconds. Start with five repetitions and increase to ten as you get stronger. Repeat the same exercise on the right side.

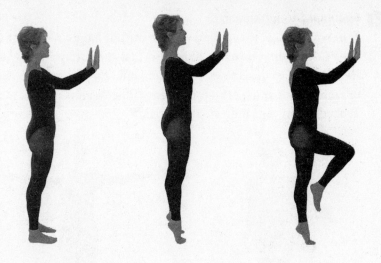

2 **Modified Knee Bend**

With your feet flat on the floor aligned with your shoulders, bend forward and put your hands on your knees. Then slowly bend your knees, keeping your hands in place until you feel your thigh muscles tighten. Hold for five seconds. Return to a standing position and bring your shoulders back, rotating your arms and hands outward so that your shoulder blades move toward each other. Start with ten repetitions and build to twenty.

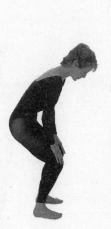
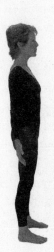

❸ Shoulder Strengthening

Start with one- or two-pound weights in your hands, with your arms at your sides. Lift your hands slowly so that they are parallel with your shoulders. Keep the elbows straight and hold for ten seconds. Start with ten repetitions and work up to twenty. The weights may be increased depending on your individual strength.

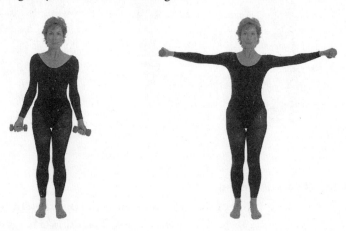

❹ Upper-Back Strengthening

Stand holding one- or two-pound weights in your hands. Bring your elbows level with your shoulders and bend them so that your fists come together. Now bring your elbows back, separating your hands so that your shoulder blades move toward each other. Hold for ten seconds and repeat ten times. Rest for a few seconds and repeat the entire exercise for a total of twenty reps.

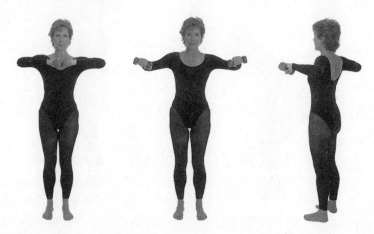

❺ Biceps and Triceps Exercises

Put your hands at your sides and hold a one- or two-pound weight in each hand. With your arm near your side, turn your left palm up, bend your elbow, and lift the weight so that your hand goes slightly behind your head and shoulder. Hold for five seconds. As you bring your arm to your side, straighten your elbow and bring the arm down straight. Repeat ten times. Then do the same thing with the right hand.

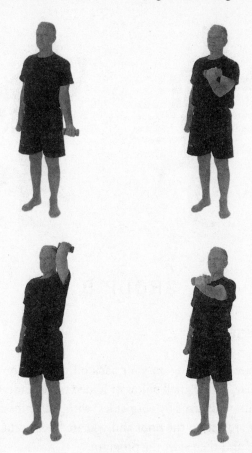

❻ Marching in Place

This simple weight-bearing exercise simulates walking or even jogging without using special equipment or leaving your home. It is a great aerobic exercise for your heart and lungs, and at the same time provides excellent weight-bearing stimulation for the bones, especially the hips, legs, and spine. It might even make you feel a little patriotic! Pumping your arms as you do this exercise is also beneficial for your heart and lungs.

Bend your elbow, make a fist, lift your knees high, and begin marching in place. Keep up a good steady pace, pushing off from your toes and swinging your arms. Do this for two minutes at first but try to build up to five minutes. You can time yourself with a kitchen timer and listen to the news or one of the morning shows on TV while you march.

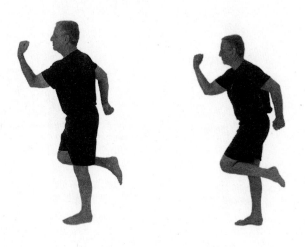

GROUP B

Floor Exercises

These exercises are done lying on your back on the floor on a comfortable rug or exercise mat, with a small pillow or folded towel under your head. Lie on your back with your arms by your sides, with your hips and knees bent so that your feet are flat on the floor and you are lying comfortably. Take a few deep breaths and then start the program.

❶ Abdominal Crunches

Place your hands on your chest. Tighten your buttocks and reach forward with your hands, lifting your head and shoulders off the floor. You should be able to bring your hands to your knees. Do not hold on to your knees, but hold this position for a slow count of ten. Slowly allow your head and shoulders to return to the floor. Repeat the exercise ten times initially but slowly build up to twenty-five repetitions. This exercise will strengthen your stomach muscles, and it is essential for the health of your back.

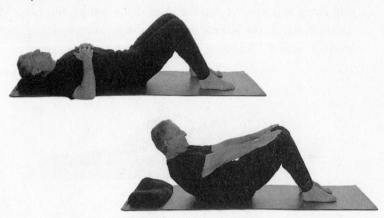

2 The Neck-to-Foot Bridge

Keeping your arms at your side, lift your hips and back off the floor with your weight on your feet and shoulders. Count to ten slowly, then return to starting position. Repeat the exercise ten times. *Caution:* If you have had any serious problem with your back, check with your doctor before doing this exercise.

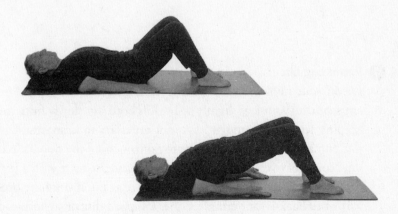

❸ Side Leg Lifts

Lie on your side, rest your head on the pillow, and put your hand behind your head. Bend your bottom knee, but keep your top knee and hip straight. Lift your top leg toward the ceiling and hold while you count to ten slowly. Repeat the exercise ten times, and then do the same exercise with the other leg while lying on the other side.

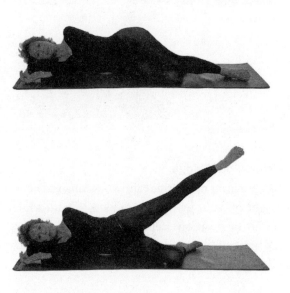

❹ Prone Leg Lift

Lie on your stomach, cross your forearms, and rest your head on your arms. Spread your legs slightly apart. Lift both legs slowly from the hips, keeping your knees straight. It is not necessary to raise your legs high, just enough so that your knees are not touching the floor. Hold for a slow count of five. This is a strenuous exercise, so start with a few repetitions and build up to ten. *Caution:* Once again, if you have problems with your back—for example, either a slipped disc or stenosis—do not try this exercise without permission from your doctor.

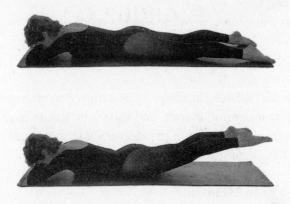

5 Prone Upper-Body Lift

Lie on your stomach and put your hands together behind your lower back or buttocks. Lift your head and shoulders from the floor and bring your shoulders back. Hold and count to five slowly. Repeat ten times. *Caution:* Again, this is a strenuous exercise, so start with a few repetitions. If you have had back problems of any sort, check with your doctor before attempting this exercise.

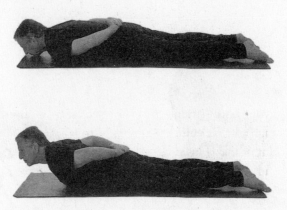

GROUP C

Sitting Exercises

These exercises are done in a chair while sitting. Any chair will do, as long as it is a sturdy one without arms. You should be able to have your hips and knees flex comfortably at a ninety-degree angle, and you should be able to rest your back against the chair.

❶ Active Knee Extension

Sit in a chair with your knee flexed at a ninety-degree angle. If you have tight hamstrings, it will be easier to do this exercise if you lean back against the chair. That will decrease the stress on your hamstrings when you extend your knee. Extend your left knee to a straight position and bring your toes back toward your face so that the toes point to the ceiling. Hold for a count of ten. Allow the foot to return to the floor and do the same with the right leg. Start with ten repetitions, alternating on each side, and progress to twenty-five. As your leg strength improves, ankle weights that vary from two to ten pounds may be added. Do this exercise slowly. It is an excellent way to strengthen your quadriceps muscles.

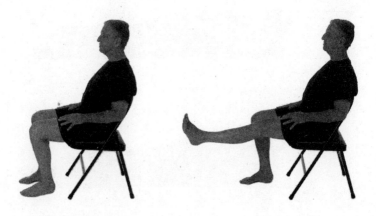

❷ Thigh Lift

This is an isometric exercise in which your muscle is tense but does not produce motion through a joint. Lift your left thigh with the left knee bent, place your hands on top of your thigh, and press down with your hand while at the same time lifting up with your thigh, resisting the pressure of your hands pushing down. Hold and count to ten slowly, and repeat on the other side. Do this exercise ten times on each side. This will help strengthen your hip flexor muscles.

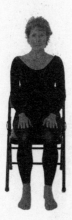 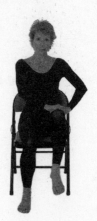

❸ Thigh-Clencher

Place a pillow between your thighs and squeeze tightly and hold while counting to ten slowly. Repeat the exercise ten times, and then repeat another ten times. This exercise strengthens your hip adductor magnus muscles.

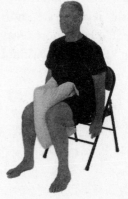

4 Thigh-Spreader

While still sitting, spread your thighs far apart. Place a hand on the outside of each thigh just above your knees. Press your hands inward as if you were pushing your thighs together, but resist the pressure, keeping your thighs apart. Hold for a count of ten. Do this ten times, rest, and repeat another ten times. This exercise strengthens your hip adductor muscles.

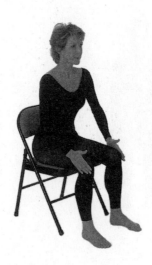

I have designed my exercise program to be quick, easy, and highly gratifying. It takes real commitment on your part, but once you get into it you'll find that the rewards are enormous. Not only will your bones become stronger, you'll have more energy, more stamina, and probably a brighter outlook on life. There is just nothing like it. Give it a try, and see for yourself.

CHAPTER TWELVE

THE SAFEST AEROBIC
AND ALTERNATIVE
THERAPIES

*Walking, Swimming, Cycling, Dancing, Yoga,
Tai Chi: Do They Help?*

A S YOU'LL NOTICE, I keep stressing the importance of stress on your bones. Let me explain why stress is so important. When we walk, for example, an electrical impulse travels up the bone every time our heel hits the ground, causing a reaction in the bone that stimulates the bone cells, strengthens the bone crystals, and improves blood flow, thereby providing the essential nutrients, including calcium, to be deposited on the bone.

Over and over again, clinical research has shown the benefits of regular exercise programs. Exercise improves the cardiovascular system, helps maintain appropriate body weight, limberness and flexibility of joints, and helps us develop strong muscles that enhance our sense of well-being, as well as our vigor and confidence. At age twenty, exercise is generally a normal accompaniment to our days, and more readily available than when we reach eighty, but the basics are the same: stretching, joint mobility, muscle strengthening, and aerobics for cardiovascular fitness and endurance. We all know that at eighty you can't do all the things you could do at twenty, but nevertheless, there are still many exercises that an eighty-year-old can do as well as a twenty-year-old. My point is that regardless of your age, you can be in better shape and health, and have stronger bones, if you exercise. Sure, there are medical problems that older people develop with time, such as various types of arthritis, back and neck maladies, and cardiovascular disorders. Despite these physical ailments, however, exercise is not only possible for older people, in my estimation it is essential.

A study that was done at the Hospital for Special Surgery found that people with osteoarthritis who walked three times a week for two months had less pain than those who didn't walk. It makes sense. Our bodies are like cars. To stay in good shape, our bodies need the right fuel (nutrition), a strong engine (good muscles), freely moving wheels and joints, a good combustion system (heart, lungs, and blood vessels), and a strong frame (bones).

Some cars are made better than others, just as some people have healthier genes than others. But even the most expensive and well-built car will not last long without proper care, while the cheapest car can run for years and many miles if it is well cared for. Each body has different endowments, some great, some not so good, but if you take care of what you have, your body will serve you well.

One of the mechanical advantages of a car is that you can replace worn and broken parts such as tires or engine parts, or even have it repainted if it starts to look dull. Many things in your body can also be replaced and fixed, but not your bones. Your frame has to last your whole lifetime, so it is imperative that you take especially good care of your bones. Good care means getting the right nutrition and the right type and amount of exercise. The first part of this book told you everything you need to know about proper nutrition. Now I'll explain which exercises are best for beautiful bones.

As an orthopedic surgeon at the Hospital for Special Surgery in New York City for more than thirty-five years, and director of the Department of Rehabilitation for thirty years, I have organized physical-training programs for patients with a multitude of orthopedic problems of varying severity, including outpatient programs for nonsurgical athletic injuries, for arthritis and neuromuscular disorders, and comprehensive programs to rehabilitate patients after surgery. In recent years, my emphasis has been on exercise programs for patients with osteopenia or osteoporosis. I have been fortunate to work with a wonderful staff at the hospital, headed by Jeme Mosca Cioppa, who is an assistant vice president at HSS and the administrative director of our rehabilitation department. *U.S. News and World Report* has always rated HHS as either number one or number two in orthopedics in the nation. I am a firm believer that knowledge and understanding are the keys to good health, and the purpose of this part of book is to provide you with knowledge of the benefits of exercise and to give you a program that is easy to understand and easy to do in a relatively short period of time. This next section will describe the more common exercises that are aerobic as well as helpful in strengthening your bones.

WALKING

Walking is the most easily available exercise to both strengthen your bones and improve your cardiovascular function. Almost anyone can walk for exercise. Exceptions are those people who suffer from spinal stenosis or other types of back disorders, people with weakness or paralysis of the lower limbs, and, rarely, those with severe circulatory impediments. Walking is a low-impact exercise and does not unduly stress your joints. At the same time, because it is weight-bearing, it strengthens your bones and helps to prevent or improve osteoporosis. Even arthritis sufferers can exercise by walking, and walking not only makes your bones stronger, it contributes greatly to your overall health and well-being.

Walking does not require much equipment. You should wear good walking shoes and dress appropriately for the weather. Comfortable clothing is the order of the day. When the temperature climbs in the summer, it is better to walk early in the morning or later in the day when the heat begins to dissipate. Walking in the boiling sun is not advisable, and can even lead to serious dehydration. Drink as much water as you can. In fact, if you walk for an hour or more, it is a good idea to take a bottle of water with you.

In the beginning, set a pace that suits you. Start with a short stride to ease the strain on your hamstring muscles. As your body grows accustomed to walking, you can lengthen your stride and increase your pace. Concentrate on keeping your body erect and breathing easily. The pace at which you walk will vary according to your general physical condition. However, the rule of thumb is that you should be able to carry on a normal conversation while you are walking. If you can't, then slow down. Eventually, your stamina will improve and you will be able to walk and talk to your heart's content.

The ideal condition for walking would be on a beautiful country road or a long, white sandy beach. Bravo for those of you who have that luxury. But one of the great things about walking is that you don't need a perfect setting in which to do it. You can use the sidewalk just outside your door, or a nearby park or schoolyard. In fact, you can use a treadmill and never leave the comfort of your home. The nice thing about a treadmill is that it's handy and not weather-dependent. Whether you walk outdoors or on a treadmill, it is important to start slowly and give your body a chance to warm up, then maintain a fairly fast pace for at least thirty minutes. Toward the end of your workout, slow your pace and allow your heart rate to gradually return to normal.

Before you start to walk, simple stretching exercises can help you avoid straining your leg muscles. Heel cords, hamstrings, and quadriceps stretch exercises are basic. Build up your endurance gradually. In the beginning, walk every other day, allowing your body to recuperate from the prior day's exercise. As your body gets stronger and your stamina improves, you can walk more often and for longer distances.

What should your goals be? I suggest you shoot for two or three miles four or five times a week. Studies have shown that if you walk three miles very fast in a half hour, or three miles more slowly in one hour, you can achieve the same cardiovascular benefits and strengthening of your bones as you would if you jogged for three miles, and you can do it with a lot less wear and tear on your feet and joints. It is essential that you walk regularly. Walking once or twice a week is helpful, but it is only a halfway measure. The minimum program should be three times a week, and five times a week is even better. Every day would be great, but most of us just can't live up to that. Three to five times a week will get you into good shape and strengthen your bones. An additional benefit of walking is that it will help flatten your belly. As you walk briskly, you unconsciously tighten your abdominal muscles, and this helps strengthen them and keep them nice and firm.

If you have had a bad hip or knee, your walking can be made easier with a cane. When I suggest the use of a cane to most of my patients, they usually respond with a "never." A cane symbolizes "oldness" to them. It is an affront to their dignity. To nullify their concern, I suggest that instead of a cane they use a "walking stick." I tell them to recall that many of the elegant gentlemen in early London carried a cane with them (although some of these canes concealed a sword). Canes or walking sticks can be extremely helpful. A cane can relieve pressure on the affected joints, and if you have a balance problem, a cane can keep you from falling. A question I'm often asked is which

What You Need for Walking

Good, comfortable shoes
Appropriate clothing
A brisk pace
Upright posture
A cane, if needed
Thirty-minute minimum, three times per week

hand to hold the cane in. The rule of thumb is that you use the cane on the opposite side of the weak or painful leg.

If you decide to use a cane, it is important to make sure the one you get is the right length for you. The handle should reach your wrist, so that the elbow is flexed only at an angle of fifteen degrees. If the cane is too low, you'll have to lean over too far, and this will strain your back. If it is too high, the flexion of your elbow will increase, and this will cause you to strain your shoulders.

Certain medical conditions may make walking for exercise inappropriate. If you have a significant back problem, circulatory problems, or abnormalities in your limbs, walking may not be right for you. Be sure to consult your doctor before beginning any exercise program.

BALANCE EXERCISES

A major problem for older people, many of whom have arthritis, is poor balance, which can cause frequent falling. Obviously, if someone has poor balance, falls frequently, and has underlying osteoporosis, the risk of fracture is great. Often, a neurological problem can result in poor balance. A simple test such as walking toe to heel, toe to heel, can help identify individuals who have a balance problem. Another way to assess your balance is to stand on one leg with your eyes open, then close your eyes and see how long you can stand like that. If you cannot stay in this position for at least ten seconds, your balance is definitely impaired. Another test is to get up from a chair, walk ten feet, and then return to a sitting position in the chair. If you have trouble doing this, there is a deficiency in your balance. Many older people are on various types of psychotropic medications that can also affect their balance and cause frequent falls. Tai chi chi is an excellent exercise for balance, and I'll discuss that later in this chapter. Meanwhile, here are some simple exercises to help improve your balance.

1. **Tandem Walking:** Walk heel to toe along an imaginary line. Try to walk at least thirty feet. Do this three times. Try it with your eyes closed for a few steps. If you are doing well, add a weight in one hand to make it more difficult.
2. **Up and Down:** Sitting in a chair with both feet on the floor, the right foot in front of the left, stand up, reverse your feet, and sit back down.

Stand up again with the left foot forward and the right foot back. Switch and sit down. This is not as easy as it sounds. Repeat ten times with each leg.

3. **Bent Knee Standing:** Stand up with both knees slightly bent. Put the weight on your right leg and abduct and lift your left leg out to the side. Try to hold this position for ten seconds. Do the same thing with the opposite leg and repeat three times.

4. **Single Leg Standing:** Stand on one leg without holding on. Try to maintain your balance for twenty seconds. To make it harder, try to do it with your eyes closed. Repeat three times on each side.

5. **Walking Backward:** Simply walk backward across the room. Try doing this on a treadmill or a hill, and you'll find out how hard it really is.

6. **Side Stepping:** Stand up and walk sideways across the room by crossing your right leg over the left leg. Then walk back across the room, crossing your left leg over your right.

If you do these six exercises regularly, you will not only improve your balance but also build your confidence, so that when you walk you will be much less likely to fall and risk breaking a bone. However, if your balance does not improve after doing these exercises for a period of time, then consider walking with a cane. Better safe than sorry, I always say.

SWIMMING

Although the buoyancy of water makes everyone feel good and allows you to exercise with little or no pain, swimming is not the best exercise to build stronger bones. It is good for cardiovascular fitness and helps build muscle. It is true that muscles that are stronger and bulkier make bone stronger, but the lack of the effect of gravity on the bones while in the water makes swimming less than ideal as an osteoporosis-prevention exercise. If you enjoy the water and swim often, chances are that you will be doing some exercises that cause a certain amount of impact. Standing in the water up to your waist

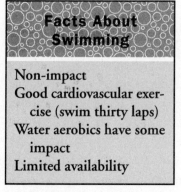

Facts About Swimming

Non-impact
Good cardiovascular exercise (swim thirty laps)
Water aerobics have some impact
Limited availability

and jumping up and down is one of them. Swinging your arms and legs in the water also causes a certain amount of impact and therefore strengthens your muscles, and this, in turn, stimulates your bones.

WATER AEROBICS

I admit that I was the first one to dismiss water aerobics as an "older person's exercise," and probably more recreational than therapeutic. However, this past summer I visited friends who invited me to participate in a water aerobics class led by a skilled instructor. What an eye-opening experience! Contrary to what I had always believed, an hour of water aerobics was as strenuous as running five miles. Our instructor, Karen Haber, had us using all of our muscles and joints, being careful to allow periods of slow activity between the more strenuous activity. The workout was superb, not only for its cardiovascular benefits and muscle strengthening, but also for its kindness to joints. Unfortunately, the availability of a pool for exercise is limited for many people. If water exercise is your thing, with a little extra effort you can locate a local Y, or a gym near your home so that you can swim all year round.

CYCLING

If you don't like to swim and you don't like to walk, there is always cycling. You can use a stationary bike indoors, or travel over the road outdoors. Cycling is an excellent exercise. By the way, if you can't use a two-wheeler outdoors, an adult three-wheel bike can provide a fine way to exercise. Once again, start slowly and increase the time and distance gradually. Hills are a special challenge that you should not attempt until you feel sufficiently strong. Choosing an outdoor bike is a serious undertaking. A bike that allows you to sit in a more upright position is the best for your back. It is all right for Lance Armstrong to race around Europe bent over his racing bike, but if you have a back problem, that position can be a source of much pain. Therefore, buy or use a bike with an upright handle. This will help take pressure off the lower back and also allow you to see ahead without straining your neck.

The seat should be comfortable for your bottom. There are different slopes and padding for the seat. Try an assortment before you make a final decision. To be the most comfortable and stress free, the distance between the handlebar and the seat should be equal to the distance between your elbow and your fingertips. The height of your seat should be adjusted so that your toes can touch the ground. If the seat is too low, it puts extra stress on your knees. Bike exercises are also great if you have had hip or knee-joint replacements. In these instances, the seat height is crucial in order to avoid excessive hip and knee flexion that is contraindicated after joint replacement. When you pedal, keep the ball of your foot, not the heel, on the pedal.

Snug pants or shorts are appropriate attire. Loose and baggy pants can get caught in the chain and cause accidents. If you are wearing loose pants, wear a clip to hold the cuffs tight around your ankle. A rearview mirror is a necessity if you ride in traffic, and a horn of some sort is useful. Always, and I mean always, obey traffic rules as if you were in a car. I shudder when I see someone on a bike go through a red light or try to weave their way through dense traffic. If you ride at dusk or at night, wear reflective clothing and have a reflector on your bike as well as headlights.

Remember, aerobic cycling is not about speed, it is about distance and time. Consistency of effort is the essential component. Again, start slowly and improve your distance gradually. Warm up with easy, steady pedaling and then increase your speed. Try to maintain an adequate speed for about twenty minutes, then slow down toward the end of your workout. If your knees are arthritic, avoid hills, although with new ten-plus speed bikes, you can still manage a hill without too much extra pressure on your knees. By pumping those pedals, you'll strengthen your leg muscles and improve your heart function and stamina. Biking is a great way to strengthen those beautiful bones.

Always wear a helmet when biking outdoors. Helmets can protect the head from serious harm in the event of an accident. I remember all too vividly a young resident at the Hospital for Special Surgery who rode his bike to work almost every day for years. One day, his bike was sideswiped by a bus, he was thrown off, and he

Tips on Cycling

Use an upright handle
Get a comfortable seat
Toes should touch the ground
The distance between the handlebar and the seat should equal the distance between your elbow and your fingertips
Obey traffic rules
Always wear a helmet

struck his head directly against the side of the curb. To compound the tragedy, a few minutes after he was hit one of his fellow residents came along and, unable to resuscitate him, had to pronounce him dead. If the young doctor had been wearing a helmet, he would be alive today.

DANCING

Dancing is not only fun, it's exercise. Even better, it's an activity that you can share with someone else. Whether it is ballroom dancing, square-dancing, the fox trot, lindy, samba, tango, or disco, you can have fun and exercise at the same time. Music is an inducement to movement. We tap our feet or clap our hands to a song. When we sing, we exercise our lungs and vocal cords. When we dance, we move our bodies and legs in concert with a specific rhythm. I envy the way disco dancers use their whole body from head to toe. They are having a ball and exercising at the same time. A good fox trot or tango is just as enjoyable, and it is a marvelous way of exercising. Dancing is a good aerobic exercise. It builds muscle strength and is weight-bearing, and so strengthens your bones. Dance classes such as ballet may be too vigorous for many people, but there are some less strenuous dance classes available. Dancing is challenging, fun, and a good way to get weight-bearing exercise.

YOGA

This time-honored exercise provides flexibility, strength, endurance, and re-laxation. Although it may look simple, the exercises you do in Yoga classes are actually quite complex. You can learn about them from a book, but it is safer to start doing them with an instructor. Many of these exercises are weight-bearing and will help strengthen your bones.

An individual instructor is nice, but not essential. I do recommend, however, that when you are starting out you don't try these exercises by yourself, that you enlist the help of a qualified instructor, whether in a class or privately. Yoga (and tai chi) classes are often held at your local Y or at a nearby health club. The Hospital for Special Surgery provides classes in Yoga and tai chi on a regular basis. The underlying principal of Yoga is to achieve maximum range of movement in all of your joints by slowly stretching your muscles and ligaments. Each position stretches a particular set of joints, and in order to maintain that position, you continuously contract your muscles. This way, Yoga builds strength more by isometric exercise than by isotonic. It also promotes inner relaxation and tranquility.

One of my patients is a well-known TV news anchor. He has always been diligent about exercise. However, he was frequently spraining a hip, or occasionally his back. It always turned out to be nothing serious, but it was very annoying for him, and these episodes would interfere with his ability to exercise. I had given him a back exercise program that helped him but did not entirely relieve his symptoms. I recently saw him again at a party, and I told him that he looked great. He explained that he had started doing Yoga six months earlier and had noticed a big difference in his body almost immediately. His flexibility had increased, he no longer had back pain or episodes of bursitis, and his stamina had improved dramatically. He also slept better. He did say, with a smile, that he was continuing to do the exercises I had prescribed for him years before.

Yoga can definitely be of great benefit to your bones and your overall health. However, if you have a serious back problem or have had a hip, shoulder, or knee replacement, many of the positions in Yoga will not be possible for you. If you have any of these problems and you want to try Yoga, you should first check with your doctor and then, if you get a green light, make sure you work with an experienced instructor who is aware of your medical condition. For most people with severe arthritic joints, Yoga is just not practical, and some positions, such as headstands, can actually be harmful and should be avoided.

TAI CHI

Tai chi, on the other hand, is an exercise everyone can do, and because it is done in a standing position, it does have a beneficial effect on your bones. Tai chi means knowing how to get to the "supreme energy." These exercises are not only beneficial, physically, but they also give you a sense of positive energy. I first became interested in tai chi many years ago when I used to jog regularly in Central Park in New York City. I would hit the road about 6:00 A.M. Part of my path was around a big reservoir. I often noticed a group of people doing tai chi in a little clearing near the track. At first I had no idea what they were doing, but I was fascinated by the grace and tranquility of their movements. I could see how relaxed yet controlled their dancelike movements were.

Then, a few years ago when I was visiting Beijing, I looked out my hotel window one morning as the sun was coming up and was amazed to see a hundred or more people, of all ages, performing the beautiful motions of tai chi. What a spectacular picture! It was like a ballet, with the sun just rising, and it is something I will always remember.

Tai chi consists of a slow, continuous, deliberate circular movement combined with deep breathing. This exercise uses all the joints and muscles in the body. It is more isotonic, but also has elements of isometric contraction, especially when a position is held for several deep breaths. Relaxation of the body and mind accompany all motions. Circulation is improved. Patients report to me that chronic pain is relieved. This exercise program is good for everyone, whether you have a bad back, have had joint replacements, or have a heart problem. Once again, I would suggest that you start out with a well-trained instructor, as you would with Yoga. Tai chi has become very popular recently, and you can find classes all over the place, especially in health clubs and local Y's. Tai chi is excellent as a weight-bearing exercise, and I highly recommend it.

TAI CHI CHI

There are many types of tai chi, and tai chi chi is one of them. It is simple, consisting of only nineteen movements, and it is easy for you to become good at it. Unlike Yoga, all tai chi chi exercises are done while standing. What's more, while you are standing you perform a mild rocking movement from your heels to your toes. This simulates walking, and thus provides stimulation that helps strengthen your bones. Although I suggest that you start out with an instructor, after just a few classes you can usually do tai chi chi on your own. It takes about twenty minutes, and you should do it every day. The combination of my exercise program and tai chi chi provides an ideal workout. Unlike Yoga, tai chi chi requires no positions that are potentially harmful.

One of my patients who was a tai chi and Yoga instructor was devastated when her bone mineral density test revealed that she had osteoporosis. Jeannette had always been careful to eat a well-balanced diet that included high-calcium foods. She was starting menopause and she was only in her mid-forties. When she began to review her medical history to try to understand why this was happening to her so early in life, she realized that her childhood diet had been very low in calcium. Therefore, when menopause occurred, her bones were already weak. She went to another doctor who suggested that she start taking Fosamax, but she didn't want to. Instead she increased the amount of calcium in her diet and began a serious weight-bearing exercise routine. She is now in her late fifties, and her bone density has returned to normal for a woman her age. She was able to reverse her condition, naturally, and today she continues to teach tai chi chi as well as work out three times a week on the NordicTrack.

OTHER ACTIVITIES

There are many other activities that can strengthen bones, including martial arts, skiing, and rowing (both with a machine and on the water). Some low-impact aerobics, such as stepping on and off a low platform, are also good, weight-bearing activities. These exercises improve cardiovascular function and have an impact on your joints, particularly your hip and knee joints. There is some aerobic equipment that does not cause impact. Examples are the StairMaster, the VersaClimber, and various elliptical trainers. Also, the NordicTrack provides one of the safest and most beneficial aerobic exercise programs, because again, there is no impact and it is done in a weight-bearing position that strengthens your bones and is great for your cardiovascular system.

Finally, I would like once again to stress the dangers of being overweight, of smoking, and of excessive alcohol or drug use. All of these conditions can cause severe damage to your bones, and if any of them apply to you, you have to subtract four points from my daily ten-point program. This means that you will have to work that much harder to keep your bones and cardiovascular system healthy. Some people may need the discipline of going to a fitness class or working with a personal trainer or physical therapist in order to stick with a regular exercise program. If you are disciplined enough to follow your own program every day, that is admirable, but if you are not then going to fitness classes or working with a personal trainer is a good, if expensive, alternative. General group classes are less expensive than a trainer, although sometimes you can find a trainer who is both well-qualified and reasonably priced.

PHYSICAL THERAPY VS. PERSONAL TRAINING

When it comes to training, many patients ask me what the difference between a trainer and a physical therapist is. For the most part trainers (often called personal trainers) become certified after studying anatomy and exercise techniques and passing an exam. They work with you on an individual basis and try to help you develop flexibility in your joints, strengthen your muscles, and build up endurance. They design and monitor an exercise routine tailored for your specific needs, and help give you the initiative to keep working toward your particular goals. Many of you think of a trainer in association with athletic teams, both collegiate and professional. These trainers are quite different from those you meet in a gym. A trainer for a professional sports team has many functions, and although he or she has an impact on an athlete's exercise program, for the most part they deal with preventing and treating injuries. These trainers take on the task of restoring injured players back to normal.

I have been fortunate enough to know and have as a close friend Ronnie Barnes, the head trainer for the NFL's New York Giants. Since 1980 Ronnie has been considered one of the best trainers in the NFL, if not in all of professional sports. He works constantly with his players. He can evaluate and differentiate between various types of athletic injuries. He can tape an ankle or a knee with the best of them. But he is also very concerned about the overall health of his athletes.

Ronnie watches the players during every practice. He continually monitors their conditioning and rehabilitation programs. When you see a player injured on the field, Ronnie will be at his side. In all of this, he works closely with the highly respected team orthopedic surgeon, Dr. Russell Warren, one of my closest colleagues at the Hospital for Special Surgery. So when you think of a personal trainer, you are thinking of a certified exercise professional (and do make sure your trainer is certified), not of a Ronnie Barnes.

A physical therapist is not a trainer, although a physical therapist can do almost anything a trainer can do. A physical therapist has a college degree and has studied biology, chemistry, zoology, anatomy, and physiology with a special emphasis on kinesiology, which is the study of muscle and joint function. Physical therapy is prescribed after an injury or surgery to any part of the musculoskeletal system. If you have had knee surgery, a physical therapist, rather than a trainer, would be instructing you and monitoring your progress. A physical therapist treats patients only with a doctor's prescription, which usually states the diagnosis for which the patient is to be treated, along with a specific exercise program.

People who are physically active, eat healthy diets rich in calcium, and have relatively low fat-to-muscle ratio will probably respond well to physical therapy, and restore their bones and muscles to health quickly.

ALTERNATIVE THERAPIES

My patients often ask me what I think of acupuncture, chiropractic treatment, and massage when it comes to preventing and treating osteoporosis. Acupuncture can be helpful in relieving some of the pain caused by osteoporosis, but chiropractic treatment should be avoided for people with osteoporosis, in my opinion. Often weak bones can't withstand the pressure of manipulation administered by a chiropractor. When you realize that a person with osteoporosis can sometimes break a rib just by sneezing or coughing, just imagine what could happen to that person after a forceful manipulation.

Massage has become very popular, and rightly so. It relaxes tight muscles, improves the flow of blood through those muscles, and relieves tension. But, since most massages are fairly vigorous, they can cause injury to a person with osteoporosis. If you have osteoporosis or osteopenia, make sure your massage therapist knows this and agrees to be very gentle with you. Also make sure that you only see licensed practitioners, and try to check their references. Often the websites of major medical centers can help you do this.

BEAUTIFUL BONES FOR LIFE

I mentioned earlier that at eighty, we can't do everything that we could at twenty. Nevertheless, getting older does not mean that you have to head for the rocking chair. It does not mean that you have to have osteoporosis and weak bones. It does not mean that your mind will not function the way it used to. Of course, there are some disorders that may limit what you are able to do and affect the quality of your life. As I look around and evaluate patients and friends, however, I see many people in their eighties and even nineties who are living happy, healthy lives. It is not all about genetics. The way you live your life plays a big role. Achievements—or a lack of them—can affect your attitude. Your family life and your friends contribute enormously to your health and well-being. You can live a long, happy, and healthy life if you are willing to start putting in the effort.

When you commit yourself to exercise and good nutrition as a way of life, you should be able to maintain your physical and mental abilities and keep your muscles strong and your bones healthy, even into your nineties. What's more, you will be able to live more vigorously and enthusiastically along the way.

It is never too late to improve your strength, agility, alertness, and the quality of your bones. That is what this book is about. Achieving this kind of improvement is my goal for you. But it is you who has to have the will, determination, and diligence to work at it. Nothing in life is free, and lately that even includes water, if you go for the bottled variety. The price you must pay for good health and strong bones that will prevent the crippling effects of osteoporosis is to eat a healthy, calcium-rich diet and exercise regularly. We all get older, but the trick is to not get old.

PART FOUR

THE
COOKBOOK

SIXTY HIGH-CALCIUM RECIPES

Table of Contents

WEIGHTS AND MEASURES 263

BREAKFAST AND LUNCHEON DISHES 264
Amazing Cheese Soufflé 264
Cheese Grits with Yogurt 265
Cheesy French Toast 266
Eggless Spinach and Mushroom Quiche 267
The Famous French Croque Monsieur Sandwich (*see Kids'
    Cookbook, p. 314*)
Sweet Onion Tart 268
Tofu Breakfast Scramble 269

SOUPS 269
Beautiful Beet and Orange Soup 269
Black Bean Soup 270
Broccoli Soup 271
Butternut Squash Soup with Tofu and Chard 272
Red Lentil Soup with Tofu and Wakame 273

SALADS AND SALAD DRESSINGS 274
Arame Salad 274
Black-eyed Pea Salad 275
Emerald Sea Salad 275
Tofu and Hijiki Salad 276
Southwestern-Style Tofu 277

Warm Spinach Salad with Blue Cheese and Almonds   278
Watercress-Walnut Salad   278
Showstopping High-Calcium Salad Dressings   279
   Buttermilk, Dill, Cucumber Dressing   279
   Blue Cheese Vinaigrette   280
   Buttermilk Blue Cheese Dressing   281

FRUITS (*can be served as desserts, too*)   281
Fresh Figs with Cream and Mint   281
Fruit Yogurt Parfait   282
Melon and Berries with Lemon-Orange Sauce   283
Roasted Figs with Goat Cheese and Almonds   284

VEGETABLES   285
Asparagus au Gratin   285
Braised Kale and Potatoes with Portobello Mushrooms   286
Broccoli and Cheese Casserole   286
Broccoli with Creamy Garlic Sauce   287
Cabbage and Cauliflower au Gratin   288
Curried Greens   289
Figs and Greens with Feta Cheese   290
Kale au Gratin   291
Mustard Greens with Raspberry Vinaigrette   292
Roasted Beets and Beet Greens with Rosemary
   Vinaigrette   292
Southern Scalloped Potatoes   293
Spicy Swiss Chard with Polenta   294
Spinach and Tofu Curry   295
Swiss Chard Supreme   296
Tasty Turnip Greens   297
Wilted Mixed Greens with Mango-Cherry Salsa   297

PASTA   298
Broccoli and Penne Pasta   298
Fettuccine Alfredo   299
Macaroni and Cheese (*see Kids' Cookbook, p. 315*)
Pasta with Sardine Sauce   300
Potato Gnocchi   301

FISH AND FISH SAUCES 302
    Baked Blue Fish with Cheese and Yogurt 302
    Trout Amandine 303
    Southern Salmon Cakes 304
    Delicious Fish Sauces 305
        Mornay Sauce 305
        Orange Sesame Sauce 306
        Pesto Sauce 306

FOUR FABULOUS SMOOTHIES (*see Kids' Cookbook p. 312*)
    Apricot Ambrosia 312
    Fresh Fruit Frosty 312
    Peanut Butter Delight 313
    Strawberry-Banana Surprise 314

Weights and Measures

1,000 micrograms	=	1 milligram
1 milligram	=	$\frac{1}{1,000}$ gram
1 ounce	=	28.35 grams
.25 pounds	=	113 grams
.50 pounds	=	227 grams
1 pound	=	16 ounces
1 pound	=	453.6 grams
1 tablespoon	=	3 teaspoons
1 tablespoon	=	½ fluid ounce
2 tablespoons	=	1 fluid ounce
1 cup	=	16 tablespoons
1 cup	=	8 fluid ounces
1 cup	=	½ pint
1 pint	=	2 cups
1 quart	=	4 cups

Breakfast and Luncheon Dishes

Amazing Cheese Soufflé

THERE IS REALLY no need to be intimidated by the thought of preparing a soufflé. A cheese soufflé is usually not as delicate as some of the others, so just follow these directions carefully and you will be "amazed" by the results. Serve this, along with a salad and some whole-grain bread, at lunch, and your guests will be singing your praises for weeks.

WHITE SAUCE
- 3 tbsp butter
- 3 tbsp flour
- 1 cup low-fat milk
- 1 small onion, studded with five or six cloves
- 1 small bay leaf
- Pinch of salt and pepper

SOUFFLÉ
- 5 tbsp grated Parmesan cheese
- 2 tbsp shredded Gruyère cheese, or Swiss cheese
- 3 egg yolks, beaten
- 4 egg whites, beaten until stiff

White Sauce:
Melt the butter in a saucepan over low heat. Add the flour and stir for about three minutes to make a roux. Slowly add the milk (you may scald the milk first for better consistency, but if you do this make sure the roux is cool before adding the milk). Add the onion and bay leaf and cook, stirring until the mixture is smooth and thick, then remove the onion and bay leaf.

Soufflé:
Prepare soufflé dish by greasing bottom of ovenproof, straight-sided dish. Butter sides generously and lightly coat with flour or grated cheese. Set aside.
Remove the white sauce from heat. Let cool for half a minute and add

the cheese and beaten egg yolks. Beat the four egg whites until stiff (but not dry) and fold the whites into the cheese mixture. Pour into a seven-inch pre-pared soufflé dish, or four individual soufflé dishes and bake for thirty min-utes in a 350°F oven. Serve immediately.

Serves four ○ **Calcium: 218 mg** ○ **Calories per serving: 226**

Basic Components: Calories 225.86; Protein 11.91 g; Carbohydrates 8.2 g; Dietary Fiber 0.16 g; Total–Fat 16.03 g; Saturated Fat 8.73 g; **Vitamins:** Vitamin B6 0.09 mg; Vitamin B12 0.77 mcg; Vitamin C 0.59 mg; Vitamin D 50.79 IU; Folate 27.67 mcg; Vitamin K 2.48 mcg; **Minerals:** Boron 0.91 mcg; Calcium 217.61 mg; Copper 0.02 mg; Magnesium 19.13 mg; Manganese 0.05 mg; Phosphorus 203.38 mg; Sodium 219.92 mg; Zinc 1.01 mg

Cheese Grits with Yogurt

COOKING GRITS in yogurt instead of water adds richness, taste, and, of course, calcium.

1½ cups plain low-fat yogurt
1 cup low-fat milk
¾ cup quick grits
2 tbsp butter
1 lemon (juice)
½ cup heavy cream
½ cup grated Parmesan cheese
½ cup grated Swiss cheese
Salt and pepper to taste

In a medium-sized saucepan bring the yogurt to a boil, gently. Add grits, stir, cover, and let return to a boil. Cook according to package direc-tions using yogurt instead of water. Stir frequently and add more liquid (milk or yogurt) if necessary. After grits are cooked, remove from heat and stir in butter, cheese, cream, and salt and pepper. Serve immediately or wrap in plastic wrap until ready to reheat and serve.

Serves four ○ **Calcium: 527 mg** ○ **Calories per serving: 439**

Basic Components: Calories 438.96; Protein 17.76 g; Carbohydrates 34.97 g; Dietary Fiber 0.52 g; Total–Fat 25.61 g; Saturated Fat 15.96 g; **Vitamins:** Vitamin B6 0.1 mg; Vitamin B12 1.14 mcg; Vitamin C 6.18 mg; Vitamin D 52.53 IU; Folate 9.17 mcg; Vitamin K 2.44 mcg; **Minerals:** Boron 0.91 mcg; Calcium 527.28 mg; Copper 0.04 mg; Magnesium 29.2 mg; Manganese 0.04 mg; Phosphorus 384.99 mg; Sodium 325.53 mg; Zinc 1.28 mg

Cheesy French Toast

THIS IS A NICE variation on the standard French toast, and it works well as a breakfast treat or as a luncheon dish when served with a salad.

TOAST
4 eggs
1 cup low-fat milk
2 tbsp low-fat sour cream
½ tsp vanilla
Pinch of salt
8 slices 12-grain bread

CHEESE MIXTURE
1 lb shredded Swiss or cheddar cheese
½ cup low-fat milk
Salt and pepper to taste
6 tbsp butter

For the French toast beat the four eggs slightly and stir in the milk, sour cream, vanilla, and a pinch of salt. Dip the bread slices into this mixture and brown in a skillet or on a well-buttered griddle. Set aside.

For the cheese mixture, place the shredded cheese, milk, salt, pepper, and butter in a saucepan over low heat, and stir. Meanwhile, place the French toast on ovenproof plates or on a greased cookie sheet and toast at 350°F for five minutes. Remove from the oven and spread the cheese mixture over the toast. Return the toast to the oven and brown lightly. Serve immediately.

Serves four (allowing two slices per person)   ○   **Calcium: 1,289 mg** ○
Calories per serving: 824

Basic Components: Calories 823.89; Protein 46.47 g; Carbohydrates 33.46 g; Dietary Fiber 3.34 g; Total–Fat 56.45 g; Saturated Fat 33.74 g; **Vitamins:** Vitamin B6 0.37 mg; Vitamin B12 2.74 mcg; Vitamin C 1.13 mg; Vitamin D 121.14 IU; Folate 74.83 mcg; Vitamin K 3.66 mcg; **Minerals:** Boron 2.03 mcg; Calcium 1,288.66 mg; Copper 0.19 mg; Magnesium 85.81 mg; Manganese 0.81 mg; Phosphorus 956.87 mg; Sodium 656.66 mg; Zinc 5.93 mg

Eggless Spinach and Mushroom Quiche

1 nine-inch unbaked pie crust

1 tbsp olive oil

1 small yellow onion, diced

2 garlic cloves, minced

1 lb baby spinach

1 cup sliced crimini mushrooms

1 tbsp fresh minced parsley

1 12-oz package low-fat silken tofu

¼ cup low-fat milk (fortified with vitamins A and D) or calcium-fortified
    soy milk

¼ tsp ground nutmeg

½ tsp white pepper

½ tsp turmeric

½ cup grated Parmesan cheese

½ cup shredded low-fat, low-sodium, or regular cheddar cheese

Preheat oven to 350°F. Bake pie crust until lightly browned. Remove from oven and set aside.

While crust is baking, heat oil in a large skillet and sauté onions and garlic until soft, about three minutes. Stir in spinach and cook for three minutes, until spinach is wilted. Add mushrooms and parsley, and cook for one minute longer. Remove from heat, pour into a large mixing bowl, and set aside.

In a food processor, combine tofu, milk, nutmeg, white pepper, turmeric and Parmesan cheese, and purée until creamy and smooth. Add to spinach mixture and stir to mix well. Transfer mixture to pie crust and bake for twenty minutes, until firm. Sprinkle cheddar cheese on top and cook for five to seven minutes longer, until cheese is melted and bubbly. Let stand for ten minutes before serving.

Serves six to eight   ○   **Calcium: 432 mg**   ○   **Calories per serving: 171**

Basic Components: Calories 170.5; Protein 12.57 g; Carbohydrates 13.7 g; Dietary Fiber 4.21 g; Total–Fat 8.7 g; Saturated Fat 2.62 g; **Vitamins:** Vitamin B6 0.09 mg; Vitamin B12 0.19 mcg; Vitamin C 12.76 mg; Vitamin D 6.23 IU; Folate 18.44 mcg; Vitamin K 4.71 mcg; **Minerals:** Boron 0.02 mcg; Calcium 431.72 mg; Copper 0.21 mg; Magnesium 27.31 mg; Manganese 0.44 mg; Phosphorus 182.05 mg; Sodium 274.78 mg; Zinc 1.2 mg

Sweet Onion Tart

THIS IS POSITIVELY delicious and easy to make if you use a preprepared pie crust. It is great for lunch or brunch with a salad and whole-grain bread.

> 2 tbsp unsalted butter (¼ stick)
> 4 cups thinly sliced sweet red onions or Vidalia onions
> 1 lemon (juice, strained)
> ½ cup dry white wine
> ⅓ cup minced fresh parsley or cilantro
> 1 prebaked tart shell (nine or ten inches)
> 2 cups shredded Swiss cheese

Preheat the oven to 450°F. Melt butter in large skillet and add onions and strained juice from one lemon. Sauté for about ten minutes. Add wine and parsley or cilantro and simmer for another fifteen minutes, being careful not to burn the onions. On the bottom of the tart shell layer half the cheese mixture, then half the onions, then the rest of the cheese and the rest of the onions. Put in the oven just long enough to melt the cheese. Be careful not to overcook this.

Serves eight   ○   **Calcium: 289 mg**   ○   **Calories per serving: 261**

Basic Components: Calories 261; Protein 9.82 g; Carbohydrates 16.74 g; Dietary Fiber 1.49 g; Total–Fat 16.44 g; Saturated Fat 8.13 g; **Vitamins:** Vitamin B6 0.11 mg; Vitamin B12 0.46 mcg; Vitamin C 9.71 mg; Vitamin D 13.84 IU; Folate 31.32 mcg; Vitamin K 14.65 mcg; **Minerals:** Boron 0.1 mcg; Calcium 288.97 mg; Copper 0.07 mg; Magnesium 21.59 mg; Manganese 0.22 mg; Phosphorus 203.69 mg; Sodium 220.31 mg; Zinc 1.28 mg

Tofu Breakfast Scramble

1 tbsp olive oil

3 medium green onions, thinly sliced

½ lb sliced button mushrooms

2 medium Roma tomatoes, diced

1 small green pepper, diced

1 12-oz package low-fat, firm silken tofu, drained and mashed

½ tsp turmeric

½ cup shredded low-fat, low-sodium, or regular cheddar cheese

In a medium skillet, heat olive oil and sauté green onions and mush-rooms until tender, about three minutes. Add tomatoes, green pepper, tofu, and turmeric, and stir to mix well. Cook for three to five minutes, or until heated through. Stir in cheese; cover pan, remove from heat, and let stand for one minute to allow cheese to melt. Season with salt and pepper, and serve immediately.

Serves four ○ **Calcium: 412 mg** ○ **Calories per serving: 149**

Basic Components: Calories 149.16; Protein 12.6 g; Carbohydrates 7.81 g; Dietary Fiber 1.96 g; Total–Fat 8.8 g; Saturated Fat 1.73 g; **Vitamins:** Vitamin B6 0.19 mg; Vitamin B12 0.14 mcg; Vitamin C 26.02 mg; Vitamin D 43.39 IU; Folate 38.13 mcg; Vitamin K 29.96 mcg; **Minerals:** Boron 3.61 mcg; Calcium 411.63 mg; Copper 0.49 mg; Magnesium 43.04 mg; Manganese 0.67 mg; Phosphorus 225.72 mg; Sodium 16.25 mg; Zinc 1.64 mg

Soups

Beautiful Beet and Orange Soup

THIS CHILLED SOUP is indeed beautiful, and very high in calcium when you use fortified orange juice. If you have any left over, just freeze it.

3 lbs beets peeled and sliced

1¼ cups chopped onions

1 tsp dried basil

1 lemon (juice, strained)

4 cups low-sodium chicken stock (you can substitute low-sodium
　　vegetable stock)

2 cups fortified orange juice

Put all ingredients except orange juice in a saucepan and simmer over medium heat for about twenty minutes, until beets are tender. Cool and purée in a blender or food processor. Add orange juice and chill. Garnish with a thin slice of lemon and a sprig of fresh basil before serving.

Serves eight　○　**Calcium: 132 mg**　○　**Calories per serving: 127**

Basic Components: Calories 127.44; Protein 5.11 g; Carbohydrates 26.3 g; Dietary Fiber 5.31 g; Total–Fat 1.11 g; Saturated Fat 0.44 g; **Vitamins:** Vitamin B6 0.18 mg; Vitamin B12 0 mcg; Vitamin C 39.74 mg; Vitamin D 0 IU; Folate 206.4 mcg; Vitamin K 5.6 mcg; **Minerals:** Boron 0.04 mcg; Calcium 131.52 mg; Copper 0.15 mg; Magnesium 42.71 mg; Manganese 0.6 mg; Phosphorus 77.5 mg; Sodium 187.39 mg; Zinc 0.66 mg

Black Bean Soup

THIS DELICIOUS STANDBY is high in calcium and refreshing any time of year. It is best when made with dried beans and topped with a teaspoon of sour cream and a sprig of dill.

1 lb dried black beans

2 quarts water

Pinch of salt

2 large onions, chopped

6 cloves minced garlic

1 tbsp olive oil

1 tsp cumin

1 lemon (juice, strained)

2 tsp oregano

2 tsp fresh dill, chopped

3 tomatoes, diced

3 scallions, chopped

½ pint low-fat sour cream

Small bunch fresh dill

Rinse the beans and place in a pot with enough water to cover them, add a pinch of salt, cover, and soak overnight. Drain beans and discard soaking water. Bring two quarts of fresh water to a boil, add beans to water, and simmer for about two hours.

Meanwhile, sauté onion and garlic in oil until lightly browned. Add cumin, lemon juice, oregano, and dill, then add this mixture to beans and cook for about another twenty minutes.

Mix the tomatoes and scallions and divide among six soup bowls. Pour in soup, garnish with sour cream and fresh dill, and serve immediately.

Serves six ○ **Calcium: 209 mg** ○ **Calories per serving: 378**

Basic Components: Calories 377.53; Protein 20.69 g; Carbohydrates 60.27 g; Dietary Fiber 13.84 g; Total–Fat 7.14 g; Saturated Fat 3.31 g; **Vitamins:** Vitamin B6 0.39 mg; Vitamin B12 0.16 mcg; Vitamin C 23.69 mg; Vitamin D 0 IU; Folate 363.71 mcg; Vitamin K 22.1 mcg; **Minerals:** Boron 1.36 mcg; Calcium 208.87 mg; Copper 0.74 mg; Magnesium 146.57 mg; Manganese 1.04 mg; Phosphorus 362.72 mg; Sodium 41.21 mg; Zinc 3.01 mg

Broccoli Soup

2 lbs broccoli

1 tbsp olive oil

1 large leek, sliced

1 tbsp flour

4 cups chicken broth

½ cup white wine

1 cup low-fat milk (fortified with vitamins A and D) or calcium-fortified
    soy milk

Pinch of nutmeg

1 cup shredded low-fat or regular Swiss cheese

Cut florets off broccoli. Peel stems and chop. Steam in a vegetable steamer until tender, about seven minutes.

While broccoli is steaming, heat olive oil and sauté leeks in a large pot until tender, about three minutes. Whisk in flour and cook for one minute. Whisk in broth and wine, and cook for two minutes, stirring occasionally. Add cooked broccoli, milk, and nutmeg, and cook for five minutes longer. In a good food processor or blender, purée until smooth. Return to pot, add cheese, and stir until melted. Season with salt and pepper, and serve hot.

Serves six ◯ **Calcium: 347 mg** ◯ **Calories per serving: 159**

Basic Components: Calories 159.18; Protein 14.47 g; Carbohydrates 13.16 g; Dietary Fiber 4.59 g; Total–Fat 5.36 g; Saturated Fat 1.88 g; **Vitamins:** Vitamin B6 0.26 mg; Vitamin B12 0.37 mcg; Vitamin C 141.24 mg; Vitamin D 17.01 IU; Folate 111.32 mcg; Vitamin K 311.21 mcg; **Minerals:** Boron 0 mcg; Calcium 346.81 mg; Copper 0.08 mg; Magnesium 48.25 mg; Manganese 0.45 mg; Phosphorus 237.42 mg; Sodium 192.69 mg; Zinc 1.49 mg

Butternut Squash Soup
with Tofu and Chard

1 tbsp olive oil

1 small yellow onion, chopped

4 large garlic cloves, minced

2 cups low-sodium chicken or vegetable broth

½ small butternut squash, peeled and cut into ½-inch cubes

1 12-oz package low-fat, firm silken tofu, drained and cubed

1 large bunch chard, trimmed and chopped

¼ cup chopped basil

½ cup freshly grated Asiago cheese

In a large, heavy pot, heat olive oil and sauté onion and garlic until onion is tender, three to five minutes. Stir in broth, squash, and tofu. Bring to a boil, reduce heat, cover, and simmer about twenty minutes, until squash is tender. In a blender or food processor, purée soup until smooth. Pour purée back into cooking pot, stir in chard and basil, and cook for three to four minutes longer, until chard is just wilted. Serve hot, topped with Asiago cheese.

Serves four   ○   **Calcium: 562 mg**   ○   **Calories per serving: 244**

Basic Components: Calories 244.09; Protein 15.78 g; Carbohydrates 22.97 g; Dietary Fiber 6.76 g; Total–Fat 12.17 g; Saturated Fat 3.87 g; **Vitamins:** Vitamin B6 0.37 mg; Vitamin B12 0.23 mcg; Vitamin C 45.01 mg; Vitamin D 5.94 IU; Folate 58.64 mcg; Vitamin K 2 mcg; **Minerals:** Boron 0.03 mcg; Calcium 562.38 mg; Copper 0.45 mg; Magnesium 162.31 mg; Manganese 1.2 mg; Phosphorus 247.82 mg; Sodium 285.29 mg; Zinc 1.81 mg

Red Lentil Soup with Tofu and Wakame

½ cup wakame
1 tbsp olive oil
1 medium yellow onion, diced
2 garlic cloves, minced
2 medium carrots, diced small
4 cups low-sodium vegetable stock
1 cup lentils
1 12-oz package low-fat, extra-firm tofu, diced
2 tbsp tamari

In a medium bowl, soak wakame in warm, filtered water until soft, about ten minutes. Drain wakame, rinse, and cut into strips, removing tough center stem. Set aside.

Heat oil in a large pot. Sauté onions, garlic, and carrots until tender, three to five minutes. Add stock and lentils; bring to a boil, reduce heat, and simmer for twenty to twenty-five minutes longer. Season with salt and pepper and serve hot.

Serves four   ○   **Calcium: 436 mg**   ○   **Calories per serving: 292**

Basic Components: Calories 292.26; Protein 22.72 g; Carbohydrates 35.92 g; Dietary Fiber 16.36 g; Total–Fat 8.04 g; Saturated Fat 1.13 g; **Vitamins:** Vitamin B6 0.39 mg; Vitamin B12 0 mcg; Vitamin C 8.28 mg; Vitamin D 0 IU; Folate 239.94 mcg; Vitamin

K 14.29 mcg; **Minerals:** Boron 0.14 mcg; Calcium 436.11 mg; Copper 0.62 mg; Magnesium 89.92 mg; Manganese 1.38 mg; Phosphorus 329.24 mg; Sodium 546.11 mg; Zinc 2.56 mg

Salads and Salad Dressings

Arame Salad

½ cup arame sea vegetable

1 cup quinoa, rinsed well

2 cups water

2 bunches scallions, sliced, including green tops

1 small red pepper, diced

1 cup fresh or frozen and thawed corn kernels

1 tbsp tamari

In a small bowl, soak arame in warm, filtered water until soft, about ten minutes. Drain and set aside.

In a medium pot, combine quinoa and water. Bring to a boil, reduce heat, cover, and simmer for fifteen minutes. Remove from heat and let stand ten minutes.

While quinoa is cooking, combine scallions, red pepper, corn, and arame in a medium bowl. Stir cooked quinoa into vegetable mixture. Add tamari and season with pepper. Serve immediately, or refrigerate for two hours to let flavors blend.

Serves four ○ **Calcium: 619 mg** ○ **Calories per serving: 212**

Basic Components: Calories 212.31; Protein 7.95 g; Carbohydrates 40.71 g; Dietary Fiber 5.22 g; Total–Fat 2.98 g; Saturated Fat 0.26 g; **Vitamins:** Vitamin B6 0.17 mg; Vitamin B12 0 mcg; Vitamin C 40.12 mg; Vitamin D 0 IU; Folate 50.53 mcg; Vitamin K 25.88 mcg; **Minerals:** Boron 0.03 mcg; Calcium 61.94 mg; Copper 0.37 mg; Magnesium 122.85 mg; Manganese 1 mg; Phosphorus 216.65 mg; Sodium 287.07 mg; Zinc 3.9 mg

Black-eyed Pea Salad

THIS GREAT SOUTHERN favorite is most delicious when served at room temperature.

1 lb dried black-eyed peas
8 cups water
Pinch of salt
1 large red onion, diced
2 medium bell peppers, diced
¾ cup sweet Champagne (or white wine)
¾ cup rice vinegar
⅔ cup olive oil
Salt and pepper to taste

Prepare the black-eyed peas according to package directions, by cooking in eight cups of lightly salted water for about forty-five minutes. Drain well and set aside to cool. When cool, mix in the onions and peppers. Whisk together the Champagne, vinegar, olive oil, salt and pepper, and stir into the black-eyed pea and pepper mixture. Serve on a bed of lettuce or watercress.

Serves eight   ○   **Calcium: 69 mg**   ○   **Calories per serving: 376**

Basic Components: Calories 376.1; Protein 13.83 g; Carbohydrates 39.05 g; Dietary Fiber 6.94 g; Total–Fat 18.8 g; Saturated Fat 2.63 g; **Vitamins:** Vitamin B6 0.3 mg; Vitamin B12 0 mcg; Vitamin C 58.63 mg; Vitamin D 0 IU; Folate 369.02 mcg; Vitamin K 12.03 mcg

Emerald Sea Salad

1 cup dried wakame
1 cup dried arame
2 tbsp rice vinegar
1 tsp toasted sesame oil
2 tbsp brown rice syrup
1 tbsp tamari
¼ cup sesame seeds

In two separate bowls, soak wakame and arame in warm, filtered water until soft, about ten minutes. Drain wakame, rinse, and cut into strips, removing tough center stem. Set aside. Drain arame, rinse, and set aside.

In a medium bowl, whisk together rice vinegar, sesame oil, rice syrup, tamari, and sesame seeds. Add sea vegetables and toss to coat. Serve immediately, or refrigerate and serve chilled.

Serves four ○ **Calcium: 77 mg** ○ **Calories per serving: 114**

Basic Components: Calories 113.75; Protein 2.71 g; Carbohydrates 15.43 g; Dietary Fiber 4.9 g; Total–Fat 5.11 g; Saturated Fat 0.73 g; **Vitamins:** Vitamin B6 0.01 mg; Vitamin B12 0 mcg; Vitamin C 0.37 mg; Vitamin D 0 IU; Folate 27.28 mcg; Vitamin K 0 mcg; **Minerals:** Boron 0 mcg; Calcium 77.06 mg; Copper 0.14 mg; Magnesium 68.38 mg; Manganese 0.25 mg; Phosphorus 69.99 mg; Sodium 392.12 mg; Zinc 5.36 mg

Tofu and Hijiki Salad

½ cup hijiki sea vegetable
¼ cup low-fat mayonnaise
1 to 2 tsp toasted sesame oil
¼ tsp white pepper
1 tsp soy sauce
1 12-oz package low-fat, firm tofu
¼ cup thinly sliced scallions
¼ cup sesame seeds

In a small bowl, soak hijiki in warm, filtered water until soft, about ten minutes. Drain and set aside.

In a medium bowl, combine mayonnaise, sesame oil, white pepper, and soy sauce; mix well to blend. Cut tofu block into three slabs; wrap each slab in a paper towel, and press to squeeze out excess water. Crumble tofu into mayonnaise. Stir in scallions, sesame seeds, and hijiki, and mix until well blended. Serve in a whole-grain pita with tomatoes and sprouts.

Serves four ○ **Calcium: 339 mg** ○ **Calories per serving: 174**

Basic Components: Calories 173.79; Protein 8.62 g; Carbohydrates 7.02 g; Dietary Fiber 3.32 g; Total–Fat 14.01 g; Saturated Fat 2.06 g; **Vitamins:** Vitamin B6 0.06 mg; Vitamin B12 0 mcg; Vitamin C 1.34 mg; Vitamin D 0 IU; Folate 24.25 mcg; Vitamin K 12.94 mcg; **Minerals:** Boron 0.01 mcg; Calcium 338.95 mg; Copper 0.29 mg; Magnesium 69.58 mg; Manganese 0.65 mg; Phosphorus 155.69 mg; Sodium 246.36 mg; Zinc 1.6 mg

Southwestern-Style Tofu

2 tbsp olive oil

1 12-oz package low-fat, extra-firm tofu

1 small yellow onion, diced

1 small green pepper, diced

1 small red pepper, diced

1 small serrano or jalapeño chili, minced, seeds removed

¾ tsp cumin

¼ to ½ tsp cayenne pepper, or to taste

1 cup corn kernels, fresh or frozen and thawed

¼ cup coarsely chopped fresh cilantro

Slice tofu block lengthwise into four slabs. Wrap each slab in a paper towel, and press to squeeze out excess water.

In a large, nonstick skillet, heat one tablespoon olive oil and fry tofu slabs until lightly browned, about five minutes on each side. Remove from pan and cut into cubes. Set aside.

In the same pan, heat remaining one tablespoon olive oil and sauté onion, green pepper, red pepper, and chili until vegetables are tender, about five minutes. Stir in cumin, cayenne pepper, corn, cilantro, and browned tofu, and heat through. Adjust seasonings, if necessary. Season with salt and pepper, and serve hot.

Serves four ○ **Calcium: 313 mg** ○ **Calories per serving: 182**

Basic Components: Calories 182.07; Protein 8.98 g; Carbohydrates 14.47 g; Dietary Fiber 2.12 g; Total–Fat 11.53 g; Saturated Fat 1.53 g; **Vitamins:** Vitamin B6 0.24 mg; Vitamin B12 0 mcg; Vitamin C 92.46 mg; Vitamin D 0 IU; Folate 48.22 mcg; Vitamin K 6.8 mcg; **Minerals:** Boron 0.03 mcg; Calcium 312.87 mg; Copper 0.22 mg; Magnesium 49.76 mg; Manganese 0.63 mg; Phosphorus 137.61 mg; Sodium 15.76 mg; Zinc 0.98 mg

Warm Spinach Salad with Blue Cheese and Almonds

8 cups baby spinach leaves

1 small red onion, thinly sliced

1 cup halved cherry tomatoes

¼ cup olive oil

2 garlic cloves, crushed

1 tbsp honey

¼ cup sherry vinegar

1 cup slivered almonds

4 oz crumbled blue cheese

Combine spinach, onion, and tomatoes in a large bowl. Set aside.

In a small saucepan, heat olive oil and garlic, and cook for one minute. Whisk in honey and sherry vinegar, and heat almost to a boil. Remove dressing from heat and pour over salad, tossing to mix. Divide greens among four plates. Sprinkle each with almonds and blue cheese, and serve immediately.

Serves four   ○   **Calcium: 261 mg**   ○   **Calories per serving: 434**

Basic Components: Calories 433.54; Protein 13.58 g; Carbohydrates 20.74 g; Dietary Fiber 6.24 g; Total–Fat 35.48 g; Saturated Fat 8.19 g; **Vitamins:** Vitamin B6 0.15 mg; Vitamin B12 0.35 mcg; Vitamin C 15.66 mg; Vitamin D 2.59 IU; Folate 27.1 mcg; Vitamin K 6.97 mcg; **Minerals:** Boron 0.66 mcg; Calcium 260.53 mg; Copper 0.36 mg; Magnesium 87.1 mg; Manganese 0.78 mg; Phosphorus 256.55 mg; Sodium 478.14 mg; Zinc 1.77 mg

Watercress-Walnut Salad

WATERCRESS IS HIGH in calcium, and so are walnuts. You can add a little blue cheese to this recipe to make a good thing even better.

1 bunch watercress, stems removed

½ cup coarsely chopped walnuts

2 oz crumbled blue cheese (optional)

Vinaigrette dressing

Wash and dry the watercress, and chop off the stems. Mix with the chopped walnuts. Add the vinaigrette dressing and sprinkle with blue cheese (if you want to) just before serving.

VINAIGRETTE DRESSING:

¼ cup balsamic vinegar

¾ cup extra-virgin olive oil

½ tsp Dijon mustard

Salt and pepper to taste

Makes one cup

Serves four ○ **Calcium: 86 mg** ○ **Calories per serving: 330**

Basic Components: Calories 339.07; Protein 6.87 g; Carbohydrates 3.38 g; Dietary Fiber 0.78 g; Total–Fat 33.93 g; Saturated Fat 6.15 g; **Vitamins:** Vitamin B6 0.11 mg; Vitamin B12 0.17 mcg; Vitamin C 0.54 mg; Vitamin D 1.3 IU; Folate 15.34 mcg; Vitamin K — mcg; **Minerals:** Boron — mcg; Calcium 86.2 mg; Copper 0.17 mg; Magnesium 34.82 mg; Manganese 0.67 mg; Phosphorus 127.36 mg; Sodium 207.32 mg; Zinc 0.91 mg

Showstopping High-Calcium Salad Dressings

Buttermilk, Dill, Cucumber Dressing

ALL OF THESE DRESSINGS go well over tomatoes, cucumbers, lettuce, arugula, and spinach.

1 cup buttermilk

2 tbsp sour cream

1 tbsp white vinegar

1 cup peeled, chopped cucumber

3 tsp fresh chopped dill

Salt and pepper to taste

Makes about 2½ cups

Combine all ingredients in a bowl and whisk well. Chill before serving.

Serves seven   ○   **Calcium: 47 mg**   ○   **Calories per serving: 31**

Basic Components: Calories 30.9; Protein 1.35 g; Carbohydrates 3.91 g; Dietary Fiber 0.12 g; Total–Fat 1.16 g; Saturated Fat 0.71 g; **Vitamins:** Vitamin B6 0.02 mg; Vitamin B12 0.09 mcg; Vitamin C 0.91 mg; Vitamin D 0.92 IU; Folate 4.57 mcg; Vitamin K 0.04 mcg; **Minerals:** Boron 0.51 mcg; Calcium 47.11 mg; Copper 0.01 mg; Magnesium 6.21 mg; Manganese 0.02 mg; Phosphorus 37.19 mg; Sodium 39.88 mg; Zinc 0.18 mg

Blue Cheese Vinaigrette

¼ cup balsamic vinegar

¾ cup extra-virgin olive oil

½ cup crumbled blue cheese

½ tsp sugar

1 lemon (juice only)

Salt and pepper to taste

Makes about 1½ cups

Whisk oil, vinegar, sugar, lemon juice, and salt and pepper together in a glass bowl. Add the crumbled blue cheese, mix, and serve.

Serves five   ○   **Calcium: 71 mg**   ○   **Calories per serving: 342**

Basic Components: Calories 342.46; Protein 2.8 g; Carbohydrates 2.46 g; Dietary Fiber 0 g; Total–Fat 35.73 g; Saturated Fat 6.88 g; **Vitamins:** Vitamin B6 0.02 mg; Vitamin B12 0.16 mcg; Vitamin C 0.06 mg; Vitamin D IU 1.18 IU; Folate 4.63 mcg; Vitamin K 0 mcg; **Minerals:** Boron 0 mcg; Calcium 71.41 mg; Copper 0.01 mg; Magnesium 2.96 mg; Manganese 0.01 mg; Phosphorus 49.76 mg; Sodium 182.34 mg; Zinc 0.34 mg

Buttermilk Blue Cheese Dressing

1 cup buttermilk
2 tbsp blue cheese
2 tbsp white-wine vinegar
1 tsp fresh lemon juice
3 tsp fresh chopped parsley
Salt and pepper to taste

Makes about 1½ cups
Mash cheese in a bowl, add other ingredients, and whisk well.

Serves five ○ **Calcium: 73 mg** ○ **Calories per serving: 32**

Basic Components: Calories 32.4; Protein 2.27 g; Carbohydrates 2.76 g; Dietary Fiber 0.02 g; Total–Fat 1.35 g; Saturated Fat 0.86 g; **Vitamins:** Vitamin B6 0.02 mg; Vitamin B12 0.14 mcg; Vitamin C 1.89 mg; Vitamin D 1.24 IU; Folate 4.61 mcg; Vitamin K 3.88 mcg; **Minerals:** Boron 0.7 mcg; Calcium 72.59 mg; Copper 0.01 mg; Magnesium 6.27 mg; Manganese 0.01 mg; Phosphorus 54.76 mg; Sodium 94.89 mg; Zinc 0.29 mg

Fruits

Fresh Figs with Cream and Mint

THIS COULDN'T BE EASIER, and it's a real treat when figs are in season.

25 small fresh figs, peeled and stemmed
2 cups heavy cream, whipped
2 tbsp sugar
1 lemon (zest)
Fresh mint

Slice each fig in half and divide among eight plates. Put heavy cream and sugar in a bowl and whip until it thickens. Top the figs with the whipped cream, a little zest from the lemon, and a sprig of mint. Serve with ginger snaps or butter cookies if you'd like.

Serves eight   O   **Calcium: 93 mg**   O   **Calories per serving: 321**

Basic Components: Calories 320.9; Protein 2.39 g; Carbohydrates 31.63 g; Dietary Fiber 5.16 g; Total–Fat 22.48 g; Saturated Fat 13.8 g; **Vitamins:** Vitamin B6 0.19 mg; Vitamin B12 0.11 mcg; Vitamin C 3.48 mg; Vitamin D 30.94 IU; Folate 11.75 mcg; Vitamin K — mcg; **Minerals:** Boron — mcg; Calcium 93.36 mg; Copper 0.11 mg; Magnesium 30.73 mg; Manganese 0.2 mg; Phosphorus 58.77 mg; Sodium 24.17 mg; Zinc 0.37 mg

Fruit Yogurt Parfait

THIS IS DELICIOUS as a luncheon dessert, or you can even try it at breakfast for a nice start to the day. You can add seedless white grapes, ripe pears, or even melon.

    1 cup plain, low-fat yogurt
    2 tbsp molasses
    3 tbsp calcium-fortified orange juice
    1 cup sliced strawberries
    1 cup sliced peaches
    ⅔ cup blueberries
    1 medium sliced banana
    ½ cup toasted, slivered almonds

Place the almonds on a cookie sheet and toast them in a 350°F oven until lightly browned, about five to ten minutes. Whisk yogurt, molasses, and orange juice together. Toss prepared fruit in a large bowl and then fill four parfait glasses or long-stem wine glasses half full with the fruit. Top with half the sauce and half the almonds. Fill glasses with remaining fruit, remaining sauce, and sprinkle remaining almonds over the top. Serve at once.

Serves four   O   **Calcium: 251 mg**   O   **Calories per serving: 207**

Basic Components: Calories 207.33; Protein 6.54 g; Carbohydrates 31.62 g; Dietary Fiber 4.36 g; Total–Fat 7.3 g; Saturated Fat 1.12 g; **Vitamins:** Vitamin B6 0.33 mg; Vitamin B12 0.32 mcg; Vitamin C 37.68 mg; Vitamin D 0.9 IU; Folate 29.8 mcg; Vitamin K 2.22 mcg; **Minerals:** Boron — mcg; Calcium 251.43 mg; Copper 0.43 mg; Magnesium 83.93 mg; Manganese 0.52 mg; Phosphorus 169.56 mg; Sodium 47.49 mg; Zinc 1.18 mg

Melon and Berries with Lemon-Orange Sauce

YOU CAN HOLLOW OUT half a watermelon in which to serve this lovely dessert if you'd like. If not, just put the fruit in parfait glasses or bowls and top with the sauce.

   ½ watermelon, cut into bite-sized pieces or made into balls
       with melon-ball scooper
   1 quart strawberries, washed and hulled
   1 quart blueberries, washed
   1 pint raspberries

SAUCE
   ⅓ cup fresh lemon juice
   ⅔ cup calcium-fortified orange juice
   ½ cup sugar
   6 egg yolks, lightly beaten together
   1½ cups heavy cream, whipped
   Grated orange peel
   Grated lemon peel
   Fresh mint for garnish

Wash, slice, and prepare the fruit and place in serving bowls or in the scooped-out watermelon shell.

To prepare the sauce, heat the lemon juice, orange juice, and sugar in a saucepan over low heat until sugar is dissolved. Put the egg yolks in a separate heavy saucepan, heat gently, and pour in the sauce, whisking constantly, until mixture is thick and smooth. Do not boil. Remove from heat and chill.

Whip the cream and fold it into the sauce, then top the fruit with the sauce and garnish with grated lemon and orange peel and a sprig of mint.

Serves ten   ○   **Calcium: 97 mg**   ○   **Calories per serving: 343**

Basic Components: Calories 342.88; Protein 4.97 g; Carbohydrates 45.34 g; Dietary Fiber 5.81 g; Total–Fat 17.85 g; Saturated Fat 9.32 g; **Vitamins:** Vitamin B6 0.46 mg; Vitamin B12 0.37 mcg; Vitamin C 81.28 mg; Vitamin D 33.3 IU; Folate 46.42 mcg; Vitamin K 1.57 mcg; **Minerals:** Boron — mcg; Calcium 96.56 mg; Copper 0.17 mg; Magnesium 42.46 mg; Manganese 0.68 mg; Phosphorus 112.32 mg; Sodium 26.69 mg; Zinc 0.82 mg

Roasted Figs with Goat Cheese and Almonds

12 fresh figs
12 oz soft goat cheese
1 cup chopped almonds

Preheat broiler. Score figs twice, lengthwise, leaving quarters attached at the base. Stuff with goat cheese and almonds. Arrange figs on a baking sheet and broil for three minutes, until cheese is bubbly and lightly browned. Serve hot.

Serves four to six   ○   **Calcium: 235 mg**   ○   **Calories per serving: 480**

Basic Components: Calories 480.87; Protein 21.79 g; Carbohydrates 33.97 g; Dietary Fiber 7.35 g; Total–Fat 30.36 g; Saturated Fat 13.45 g; **Vitamins:** Vitamin B6 0.41 mg; Vitamin B12 0.16 mcg; Vitamin C 3 mg; Vitamin D 5.43 IU; Folate 28.91 mcg; Vitamin K — mcg; **Minerals:** Boron — mcg; Calcium 235.49 mg; Copper 0.97 mg; Magnesium 109.84 mg; Manganese 0.28 mg; Phosphorus 363.75 mg; Sodium 314.48 mg; Zinc 1.77 mg

Vegetables

Asparagus au Gratin

NOTHING COULD BE EASIER or healthier than this simple, elegant way of serving fresh asparagus. It is especially delightful in the spring when you can find the fresh, thin asparagus stalks.

    1 lb asparagus, trimmed
    1 lemon (juice)
    8 tbsp heavy cream
    ½ cup grated sharp cheddar cheese
    ½ cup grated Swiss cheese

Cut off the tough ends of the asparagus and discard. Peel the stems with a sharp knife or vegetable peeler. Steam the asparagus in a covered steamer in two inches of water, until just tender, about three to five minutes. Remove from heat, drain, place on ovenproof baking dish, and squeeze juice of one lemon over the asparagus. Pour the cream over the asparagus tips and then sprinkle the mixed grated cheeses over the tips. Run under the broiler for a few seconds, until the cheese starts to melt and brown. Serve immediately.

Serves four ○ **Calcium: 276** ○ **Calories per serving: 239**

Basic Components: Calories 239.31; Protein 10.6 g; Carbohydrates 7.63 g; Dietary Fiber 2.43 g; Total–Fat 19.62 g; Saturated Fat 12.28 g; **Vitamins:** Vitamin B6 0.18 mg; Vitamin B12 0.4 mcg; Vitamin C 20.55 mg; Vitamin D 23.11 IU; Folate 151.28 mcg; Vitamin K 45.78 mcg; **Minerals:** Boron — mcg; Calcium 275.54 mg; Copper 0.21 mg; Magnesium 32 mg; Manganese 0.3 mg; Phosphorus 236.6 mg; Sodium 136.51 mg; Zinc 1.56 mg

Braised Kale and Potatoes with Portobello Mushrooms

4 small red potatoes, cubed

1 tbsp olive oil

1 cup portobello mushrooms, chopped

1 small red onion, diced

4 garlic cloves, minced

1 pound kale, trimmed and chopped

Boil potatoes in a medium pot with a tight-fitting lid until just tender, seven to ten minutes. Drain and set aside.

Heat oil in a medium skillet and sauté mushrooms, onions, and garlic for three minutes. Add cooked potatoes and sauté until potatoes are lightly browned and mushrooms are tender, three to five minutes. Add kale with water still clinging to the leaves; cover skillet and cook for two to four minutes, until kale is bright green and tender. Season with salt and pepper, and serve hot.

Serves four   ○   **Calcium: 181 mg**   ○   **Calories per serving: 228**

Basic Components: Calories 227.5; Protein 8.06 g; Carbohydrates 42.34 g; Dietary Fiber 5.96 g; Total–Fat 4.51 g; Saturated Fat 0.62 g; **Vitamins:** Vitamin B6 0.68 mg; Vitamin B12 0.01 mcg; Vitamin C 171.65 mg; Vitamin D 0 IU; Folate 73.16 mcg; Vitamin K 928.48 mcg; **Minerals:** Boron 0.03 mcg; Calcium 181.3 mg; Copper 0.69 mg; Magnesium 81.6 mg; Manganese 1.23 mg; Phosphorus 214.52 mg; Sodium 61.7 mg; Zinc 1.3 mg

Broccoli and Cheese Casserole

1 tbsp olive oil

1 small yellow onion, diced

4 garlic cloves, minced

1 tbsp flour

1 cup low-fat milk or calcium-fortified soy milk

½ cup low-sodium chicken stock

2 cups broccoli florets

1 cup shredded low-fat or regular cheddar cheese

3 cups cooked brown rice

Preheat oven to 325°F.

In a large skillet, heat olive oil and sauté onion and garlic for three minutes, until onion is just tender. Whisk in flour and cook for one minute, whisking constantly. Whisk in soy milk and stock and cook until thick and smooth. Stir in broccoli and cheese, and season with salt and pepper.

Place rice in a lightly oiled eight-inch square baking dish. Pour broccoli mixture over rice and bake, uncovered, for twenty-five to thirty minutes, until broccoli is tender and cheese is bubbly. Let stand for five minutes before serving.

Serves six to eight ○ **Calcium: 157 mg** ○ **Calories per serving: 200**

Basic Components: Calories 199.8; Protein 9.95 g; Carbohydrates 28.82 g; Dietary Fiber 2.72 g; Total–Fat 5.1 g; Saturated Fat 1.63 g; **Vitamins:** Vitamin B6 0.23 mg; Vitamin B12 0.09 mcg; Vitamin C 23.63 mg; Vitamin D 16.67 IU; Folate 26.72 mcg; Vitamin K 1.34 mcg; **Minerals:** Boron 0.02 mcg; Calcium 156.5 mg; Copper 0.13 mg; Magnesium 52.52 mg; Manganese 0.99 mg; Phosphorus 194.63 mg; Sodium 157.86 mg; Zinc 1.1 mg

Broccoli with Creamy Garlic Sauce

1 large head broccoli, washed well

1 tbsp olive oil

4 medium garlic cloves, crushed

1 tbsp flour

1 cup low-fat milk (fortified with vitamins A and D)
    or calcium-fortified soy milk

¼ tsp white pepper

Cut lower stems off broccoli and set aside. Slice broccoli tops lengthwise. Peel stems and slice into strips. Place a vegetable steamer in a medium saucepan with a tight-fitting lid, and steam broccoli until bright green and just tender, five to seven minutes.

While broccoli is steaming, heat olive oil in a medium saucepan. Sauté garlic until just tender, about three minutes. Whisk in flour and cook on low heat for one minute. Whisk in soy milk and white pepper; cook over low heat for three to five minutes longer, or until sauce is thick and bubbly. Season with salt.

Remove broccoli from steamer and arrange on a serving platter. Drizzle with sauce and serve hot as a side dish.

Serves four ○ **Calcium: 159 mg** ○ **Calories per serving: 117**

Basic Components: Calories 116.99; Protein 7.73 g; Carbohydrates 14.44 g; Dietary Fiber 5.09 g; Total–Fat 4.63 g; Saturated Fat 0.93 g; **Vitamins:** Vitamin B6 0.28 mg; Vitamin B12 0 mcg; Vitamin C 128.16 mg; Vitamin D 25 IU; Folate 88.16 mcg; Vitamin K 460.94 mcg; **Minerals:** Boron — mcg; Calcium 159.37 mg; Copper 0.09 mg; Magnesium 42.14 mg; Manganese 0.44 mg; Phosphorus 107.36 mg; Sodium 77.28 mg; Zinc 0.7 mg

Cabbage and Cauliflower au Gratin

THIS DELICIOUS DISH can be made with celery and Swiss chard, cabbage, and/or cauliflower, mixed two at a time, or separately.

    2 cups coarsely shredded fresh green cabbage
    2 cups cauliflower, chopped
    2 cups cheese sauce
    ¾ cup lightly toasted and buttered bread crumbs
    ⅔ cup grated Swiss cheese or Swiss and cheddar mixed
        Cheese sauce
    4 tbsp butter
    3 tbsp flour
    2 cups low-fat milk
    ½ cup grated Swiss cheese (or half Parmesan and half Swiss cheese)
    Salt and pepper to taste

Heat oven to 375°F. Place cabbage and cauliflower in a pot of lightly salted boiling water and cook for about eight minutes, until tender. Drain well and put vegetables in casserole. Spoon the sauce over the vegetables. Mix bread crumbs and cheese and spread over the top. Bake twenty-five to thirty minutes until crumbs are light brown.

Prepare the cheese sauce by melting butter in a heavy saucepan and add flour and whisk well. Gradually add milk and heat slowly until milk has thickened, about two minutes. Add cheese, salt and pepper, and stir until melted completely.

Serves six ○ **Calcium: 320 mg** ○ **Calories per serving: 236**

Basic Components: Calories 236.14; Protein 10.74 g; Carbohydrates 19.23 g; Dietary Fiber 1.81 g; Total–Fat 13.08 g; Saturated Fat 7.94 g; **Vitamins:** Vitamin B6 0.13 mg; Vitamin B12 0.58 mcg; Vitamin C 27.93 mg; Vitamin D 41.47 IU; Folate 43.53 mcg; Vitamin K 4.36 mcg; **Minerals:** Boron 1.05 mcg; Calcium 320.02 mg; Copper 0.06 mg; Magnesium 28.26 mg; Manganese 0.19 mg; Phosphorus 221.22 mg; Sodium 217.04 mg; Zinc 1.3 mg

Curried Greens

1 tbsp olive oil
1 medium yellow onion, diced
2 garlic cloves, minced
1 to 2 tsp red curry paste
1 cup low-sodium chicken stock
½ lb turnip greens, trimmed and chopped
½ lb collard greens, trimmed and chopped
½ lb kale, trimmed and chopped

Heat oil in a medium pot. Sauté onion and garlic until onion is just tender, two to three minutes. In a small bowl, combine curry paste and stock, and blend until smooth. Add mixture to pot and bring to a boil. Add greens, reduce heat, cover, and cook until just tender, three to four minutes. Serve hot over brown rice.

Serves four ○ **Calcium: 279 mg** ○ **Calories per serving: 112**

Basic Components: Calories 111.71; Protein 5.29 g; Carbohydrates 15.57 g; Dietary Fiber 5.52 g; Total–Fat 4.62 g; Saturated Fat 0.78 g; **Vitamins:** Vitamin B6 0.45 mg; Vitamin B12 0 mcg; Vitamin C 124.3 mg; Vitamin D 0 IU; Folate 225.83 mcg; Vitamin K 607.76 mcg; **Minerals:** Boron 0.05 mcg; Calcium 278.55 mg; Copper 0.41 mg; Magnesium 45.08 mg; Manganese 0.92 mg; Phosphorus 72.64 mg; Sodium 108.9 mg; Zinc 0.5 mg

Figs and Greens with Feta Cheese

2 tsp Dijon mustard
1 tbsp fresh thyme leaves
¼ cup balsamic vinegar
¼ cup olive oil
4 cups spinach
4 cups arugula
16 fresh figs, halved
½ cup feta cheese
¼ cup toasted slivered almonds

In a small bowl, combine mustard, thyme, and vinegar. Whisk in olive oil until thickened. In a medium bowl, toss together spinach and arugula. Drizzle with vinaigrette and toss to coat. Divide greens among four individual plates. Arrange four figs on each plate. Drizzle figs with remaining vinaigrette, sprinkle with feta cheese and almonds, and serve.

Serves four   ◯   **Calcium: 265 mg**   ◯   **Calories per serving: 433**

Basic Components: Calories 433; Protein 7.45 g; Carbohydrates 58.48 g; Dietary Fiber 10.46 g; Total–Fat 21.92 g; Saturated Fat 5.08 g; **Vitamins:** Vitamin B6 0.45 mg; Vitamin B12 0.32 mcg; Vitamin C 17.59 mg; Vitamin D 3.75 IU; Folate 101.19 mcg; Vitamin K 126.61 mcg; **Minerals:** Boron — mcg; Calcium 264.71 mg; Copper 0.32 mg; Magnesium 99.71 mg; Manganese 0.85 mg; Phosphorus 159.8 mg; Sodium 304.03 mg; Zinc 1.42 mg

Kale au Gratin

1½ lbs kale, trimmed and chopped

2 tbsp olive oil

2 large garlic cloves, minced

3 large eggs, beaten

1 cup low-fat milk (fortified with vitamins A and D)
   or calcium-fortified soy milk

¼ tsp white pepper

½ tsp salt

½ cup shredded Parmesan cheese

½ cup whole-grain bread crumbs

Preheat oven to 375°F.

Cook kale in a large pot of boiling, salted water for two minutes. Drain and rinse with cold water. Set aside.

In a large, nonstick skillet, heat one tablespoon olive oil and sauté garlic for one minute. Add greens and stir to coat.

In a small bowl, beat together eggs, milk, white pepper, and salt. Stir in greens and cheese. Transfer to a lightly oiled eight-inch square baking dish. Top with bread crumbs and drizzle with remaining oil. Bake for forty minutes, until browned and firm. Remove from oven and let stand for five minutes before serving.

Serves four   ○   **Calcium: 386 mg**   ○   **Calories per serving: 306**

Basic Components: Calories 305.77; Protein 16.66 g; Carbohydrates 30.83 g; Dietary Fiber 3.97 g; Total–Fat 14.58 g; Saturated Fat 3.61 g; **Vitamins:** Vitamin B6 0.53 mg; Vitamin B12 0.38 mcg; Vitamin C 204.92 mg; Vitamin D 44.5 IU; Folate 67.01 mcg; Vitamin K 1,393.02 mcg; **Minerals:** Boron 0.56 mcg; Calcium 386.3 mg; Copper 0.5 mg; Magnesium 62.1 mg; Manganese 1.36 mg; Phosphorus 204.63 mg; Sodium 623.84 mg; Zinc 1.18 mg

Mustard Greens with Raspberry Vinaigrette

1½ lbs young mustard greens, trimmed and coarsely chopped

2 tbsp white-wine vinegar

2 tbsp olive oil

2 tbsp raspberry preserves

Bring a medium pot of salted water to a boil. Add greens and cook for two minutes, until just wilted. Drain greens and plunge into cold water to stop cooking. Drain and let cool, refrigerated, for forty-five minutes. While greens are cooling, whisk together in a medium bowl vinegar, olive oil, and raspberry preserves. Add cooled greens and toss to coat. Serve immediately.

Serves four   ○   **Calcium: 175 mg**   ○   **Calories per serving: 131**

Basic Components: Calories 131.4; Protein 4.59 g; Carbohydrates 15.33 g; Dietary Fiber 5.61 g; Total–Fat 7.09 g; Saturated Fat 0.93 g; **Vitamins:** Vitamin B6 0.31 mg; Vitamin B12 0 mcg; Vitamin C 119.67 mg; Vitamin D 0 IU; Folate 318.09 mcg; Vitamin K 292.48 mcg; **Minerals:** Boron — mcg; Calcium 175.2 mg; Copper 0.25 mg; Magnesium 54.43 mg; Manganese 0.82 mg; Phosphorus 73.21 mg; Sodium 42.53 mg; Zinc 0.34 mg

Roasted Beets and Beet Greens with Rosemary Vinaigrette

¼ cup plus 1 tbsp olive oil

1 lb beets, peeled, cut into ½-inch pieces

2 tsp Dijon mustard

1 garlic clove, finely minced

1 tbsp minced fresh rosemary

2 tbsp sherry vinegar

8 cups beet greens, washed and trimmed

Preheat oven to 400°F.

In a large bowl, toss together beets and one tablespoon olive oil. Toss to coat well, and season well with salt and pepper. Transfer to a baking sheet, cover loosely with foil, and roast for thirty to thirty-five minutes, stirring occasionally, until tender.

While beets are roasting, combine mustard, garlic, rosemary, and vinegar in a small bowl. In a slow, steady stream, whisk in remaining olive oil. Set aside.

Heat a large skillet over medium-high heat. Place beet greens with water still clinging to the leaves in the skillet. Cover and cook for two minutes, or until just wilted. Stir in cooked beets; drizzle with vinaigrette and toss to coat. Serve immediately.

Serves four ○ **Calcium: 112 mg** ○ **Calories per serving: 219**

Basic Components: Calories 219.31; Protein 3.3 g; Carbohydrates 14.99 g; Dietary Fiber 6.08 g; Total–Fat 17.15 g; Saturated Fat 2.33 g; **Vitamins:** Vitamin B6 0.17 mg; Vitamin B12 0 mcg; Vitamin C 28.74 mg; Vitamin D 0 IU; Folate 135.6 mcg; Vitamin K 11.67 mcg; **Minerals:** Boron — mcg; Calcium 112.21 mg; Copper 0.23 mg; Magnesium 81.47 mg; Manganese 0.69 mg; Phosphorus 78.17 mg; Sodium 301.93 mg; Zinc 0.71 mg

Southern Scalloped Potatoes

THIS SUMPTUOUS SOUTHERN FAVORITE is high in calcium and delicious with any hearty fall or winter meal.

6 cups boiling potatoes, thinly sliced (⅛ inch thick)
1 clove garlic
½ stick (4 tbsp) unsalted butter
Dash of salt and pepper
1½ cups grated Swiss cheese
1 cup low-fat milk

Preheat oven to 425°F. Peel and slice potatoes and put slices in a bowl of ice water until ready to use. Rub a ten-inch baking dish with the garlic clove and then grease it generously with butter. Drain the potato slices and pat dry, removing as much water as possible. Layer them in a dish and divide alternately with the butter, salt and pepper, and cheese, saving a layer of cheese for the top. Place in the oven and bake for about thirty-five minutes, until top is lightly browned and you can pierce the potatoes with a knife.

Serves eight   O   **Calcium: 239 mg**   O   **Calories per serving: 224**

Basic Components: Calories 224.7; Protein 8.64 g; Carbohydrates 22 g; Dietary Fiber 1.38 g; Total–Fat 11.65 g; Saturated Fat 7.36 g; **Vitamins:** Vitamin B6 0.31 mg; Vitamin B12 0.46 mcg; Vitamin C 12.12 mg; Vitamin D 25.03 IU; Folate 11.31 mcg; Vitamin K 1.22 mcg; **Minerals:** Boron 0.46 mcg; Calcium 239.03 mg; Copper 0.21 mg; Magnesium 34.6 mg; Manganese 0.16 mg; Phosphorus 199.71 mg; Sodium 73.46 mg; Zinc 1.18 mg

Spicy Swiss Chard with Polenta

3 cups low-sodium chicken broth
2 cups low-fat milk (fortified with vitamins A and D)
1 cup polenta
1 tbsp olive oil
4 garlic cloves, peeled and chopped
½ to 1 tsp red pepper flakes
1 large bunch Swiss chard, trimmed and coarsely chopped
1 cup shredded Parmesan or romano cheese
Additional cheese for serving, if desired

In a medium pot, whisk together broth, milk, and polenta. Bring to a boil, continuing to whisk. Reduce heat to low and cook, stirring frequently, until polenta is smooth and cooked through, about fifteen minutes.

While polenta is cooking, heat oil in a large skillet over medium-high heat and sauté garlic and red pepper flakes for one minute. Add greens with water still clinging to the leaves; cover, reduce heat, and let greens steam for three minutes, or until wilted.

Whisk cheese into cooked polenta and stir to mix. Divide polenta among four bowls and top each with greens. Sprinkle with additional cheese, if desired, and serve immediately.

Serves four   O   **Calcium: 477 mg**   O   **Calories per serving: 376**

Basic Components: Calories 376.1; Protein 20.51 g; Carbohydrates 49.61 g; Dietary Fiber 6.24 g; Total–Fat 11.35 g; Saturated Fat 5.27 g; **Vitamins:** Vitamin B6 0.15 mg; Vitamin B12 0.28 mcg; Vitamin C 20.13 mg; Vitamin D 55.6 IU; Folate 11 mcg; Vitamin K 1.65 mcg; **Minerals:** Boron — mcg; Calcium 477.46 mg; Copper 0.18 mg; Magnesium 99.73 mg; Manganese 0.4 mg; Phosphorus 185.75 mg; Sodium 670.2 mg; Zinc 1.02 mg

Spinach and Tofu Curry

1 can light coconut milk
2 tbsp green Thai curry paste
1½ cups low-sodium chicken stock
2 tbsp fish sauce
1 tbsp honey
3 lime leaves
3 lemongrass stalks, cut into thirds and crushed with a knife
3 ¼-inch slices galangal (Thai ginger)
1 lb low-fat, extra-firm tofu, cubed
1 medium red pepper, cut into chunks
1 small yellow onion, cut into chunks
8 cups baby spinach leaves
¼ cup coarsely chopped fresh Thai or sweet basil
Additional basil for garnish

In a large saucepan, whisk together coconut milk and curry paste. Whisk in chicken stock, fish sauce, and honey. Add lime leaves, lemongrass, and ginger. Bring to a boil. Add tofu, red pepper, and onion, and cook over medium heat until pepper is tender (about ten minutes). Remove lemongrass, lime leaves, and ginger slices. Stir in spinach and basil, and cook for one to two minutes longer, or until spinach is just wilted. Serve hot over basmati rice with additional whole basil leaves as garnish.

Serves four to six   ○   **Calcium: 451 mg**   ○   **Calories per serving: 205**

Basic Components: Calories 205.21; Protein 13.53 g; Carbohydrates 20.27 g; Dietary Fiber 3.65 g; Total–Fat 10.35 g; Saturated Fat 5.07 g; **Vitamins:** Vitamin B6 0.19 mg; Vitamin B12 0.04 mcg; Vitamin C 65.16 mg; Vitamin D 0 IU; Folate 33.27 mcg; Vitamin K 0.35 mcg; **Minerals:** Boron 0.03 mcg; Calcium 451.4 mg; Copper 0.26 mg; Magnesium 56.75 mg; Manganese 0.81 mg; Phosphorus 124.1 mg; Sodium 956.7 mg; Zinc 1.03 mg

Swiss Chard Supreme

SWISS CHARD MAY SOUND A LITTLE EXOTIC, especially if you are not from the South, but it really isn't. You can find it in grocery stores everywhere, and it is a fine source of calcium and other nutrients provided by green, leafy vegetables. This recipe is particularly good if you use both the green and red variety, but two batches of either one will do just fine.

    2 bunches Swiss chard (preferably one green and one red)
    1 lemon
    2 tbsp olive oil
    1 medium onion, peeled and chopped
    1½ tbsp whole sesame seeds
    1 tbsp sugar
    1 tbsp brown-rice vinegar (or white vinegar)

Wash the chard carefully and slice the leafy part into one-and-a-half-inch strips. Discard the stems. Place the chard in a steamer or saucepan with two inches of water, cover, and steam for twenty minutes.

Meanwhile, peel and chop the onion and sauté it in the olive oil over low heat, making sure the onions become clear but not burned. Stir in sesame seeds, sugar, juice of one lemon (strained to eliminate seeds), and vinegar. Sauté the mixture for one minute. When the chard is ready, drain it, toss with the onion mixture, and serve.

Serves four   ○   **Calcium: 153 mg**   ○   **Calories per serving: 148**

Basic Components: Calories 147.63; Protein 4.97 g; Carbohydrates 16.26 g; Dietary Fiber 4.61 g; Total–Fat 8.74 g; Saturated Fat 1.2 g; **Vitamins:** Vitamin B6 0.29 mg; Vitamin B12 0 mcg; Vitamin C 75.22 mg; Vitamin D 0 IU; Folate 41.56 mcg; Vitamin K 1,886.3 mcg; **Minerals:** Boron 0.05 mcg; Calcium 152.9 mg; Copper 0.5 mg; Magnesium 198.26 mg; Manganese 0.95 mg; Phosphorus 134.17 mg; Sodium 484.59 mg; Zinc 1.1 mg

Tasty Turnip Greens

THIS DELICIOUS, high-calcium recipe can also be made without the bacon if you are a vegetarian.

6 bunches turnip greens
5 slices bacon
2 tbsp brown sugar
Dash of salt and pepper
½ cup water
2 tbsp vinegar

Take the leaves from the stems and discard the stems. Wash the leaves carefully. Slice the bacon into one-inch strips and cook it in a skillet for seven or eight minutes until translucent. Add turnip green leaves to the skillet, along with sugar, seasoning, and water. Stir the mixture and allow to simmer over very low heat for about two and a half hours. Remove from the liquid with a slotted spoon and serve.

Serves eight   ○   **Calcium: 219 mg**   ○   **Calories per serving: 123**

Basic Components: Calories 122.76; Protein 2.93 g; Carbohydrates 10.04 g; Dietary Fiber 3.63 g; Total–Fat 8.49 g; Saturated Fat 3.09 g; **Vitamins:** Vitamin B6 0.32 mg; Vitamin B12 0.13 mcg; Vitamin C 68.04 mg; Vitamin D 0 IU; Folate 220.31 mcg; Vitamin K 284.63 mcg; **Minerals:** Boron — mcg; Calcium 219.37 mg; Copper 0.42 mg; Magnesium 37.43 mg; Manganese 0.54 mg; Phosphorus 68.5 mg; Sodium 150.15 mg; Zinc 0.38 mg

Wilted Mixed Greens
with Mango-Cherry Salsa

1 cup chopped mango, fresh or frozen and thawed
1 cup chopped cherries, fresh or frozen and thawed
1 medium serrano or jalapeño pepper, minced
¼ cup finely chopped green onion

¼ cup chopped fresh cilantro

1 tbsp fresh lime juice

2 lbs mixed greens (young kale, chard, spinach, mustard greens)

In a medium bowl, combine mango, cherries, chili pepper, green onion, cilantro, and lime. Stir to mix, and season with salt and pepper. Refrigerate for two hours.

Heat a large skillet over medium-high heat. Add greens with water still clinging to the leaves; cover, reduce heat, and cook until greens are wilted, three to four minutes. Remove from heat and plunge into cold water to stop cooking. Drain well and refrigerate for thirty minutes to chill. Divide greens among four individual plates and spoon salsa over each plate. Serve immediately.

Serves four   ○   **Calcium: 237 mg**   ○   **Calories per serving: 123**

Basic Components: Calories 123.47; Protein 6.91 g; Carbohydrates 26.6 g; Dietary Fiber 7.33 g; Total–Fat 1.32 g; Saturated Fat 0.22 g; **Vitamins:** Vitamin B6 0.51 mg; Vitamin B12 0 mcg; Vitamin C 158.64 mg; Vitamin D 0 IU; Folate 254.07 mcg; Vitamin K 1,269.98 mcg; **Minerals:** Boron 0.01 mcg; Calcium 236.5 mg; Copper 0.52 mg; Magnesium 138.41 mg; Manganese 1.5 mg; Phosphorus 126.17 mg; Sodium 207.69 mg; Zinc 0.94 mg

Pasta

Broccoli and Penne Pasta

8 oz dry penne pasta

2 cups low-fat milk

1 tbsp butter

1 oz tomato sauce

½ cup white wine

4 garlic cloves, minced

1 cup broccoli florets

½ cup fresh sliced mushrooms
½ cup grated romano cheese

Cook pasta in a large pot of boiling, salted water until tender but firm to the bite (ten to twelve minutes). Drain and return to pot.

While pasta is cooking, combine milk, butter, tomato sauce, wine, garlic, broccoli, and mushrooms in a medium pot. Cook over medium heat for about five minutes, or until broccoli is just tender. Add sauce to drained pasta and toss to coat. Stir in romano cheese, stir to mix, and serve immediately.

Serves four ○ **Calcium: 312 mg** ○ **Calories per serving: 374**

Basic Components: Calories 373.55; Protein 16.94 g; Carbohydrates 52.46 g; Dietary Fiber 2.18 g; Total–Fat 8.5 g; Saturated Fat 4.81 g; **Vitamins:** Vitamin B6 0.16 mg; Vitamin B12 0.15 mcg; Vitamin C 19.88 mg; Vitamin D 62.09 IU; Folate 146.7 mcg; Vitamin K 0 mcg; **Minerals:** Boron 0.65 mcg; Calcium 311.93 mg; Copper 0.23 mg; Magnesium 43.16 mg; Manganese 0.65 mg; Phosphorus 216.75 mg; Sodium 227.67 mg; Zinc 1.24 mg

Fettuccine Alfredo

THIS FAMOUS PASTA DISH is high in calcium, but because of the cream, it is somewhat high in fat, too. It is delicious, easy to make, and tastes best when made with the fresh pasta that you can buy everywhere now.

THE SAUCE

2 oz butter
1 cup freshly grated Parmesan cheese
1 cup cream
¼ cup finely chopped parsley
Freshly ground white pepper
Pinch of nutmeg

THE PASTA

10 oz fettuccine, preferably fresh

Prepare the pasta according to package directions and set aside. Melt butter in a large saucepan and quickly swirl the pasta through it. Add the cheese and toss with forks. Pour the room temperature cream on top and mix well. Season with salt, pepper, and nutmeg, top with parsley, and serve immediately.

Serves four ○ **Calcium: 335 mg** ○ **Calories per serving: 657**

Basic Components: Calories 657.3; Protein 19.4 g; Carbohydrates 55.45 g; Dietary Fiber 2.36 g; Total–Fat 40.54 g; Saturated Fat 24.97 g; **Vitamins:** Vitamin B6 0.04 mg; Vitamin B12 0.41 mcg; Vitamin C 5.35 mg; Vitamin D 44.48 IU; Folate 161.78 mcg; Vitamin K 20.25 mcg; **Minerals:** Boron — mcg; Calcium 335.2 mg; Copper 0.2 mg; Magnesium 54.61 mg; Manganese 0.01 mg; Phosphorus 303.59 mg; Sodium 402.1 mg; Zinc 1.64 mg

Pasta with Sardine Sauce

THIS IS A SOUTHERN ITALIAN RECIPE, originally from Palermo, in Sicily. You can use it with any kind of tube pasta, and it is a great way to take advantage of the generous amount of calcium in sardines.

1 lb pasta
1 small head fresh fennel
4½ cups water
1 medium onion
2 anchovy fillets (optional)
1 lb canned sardines
⅓ cup pine nuts
1 tbsp olive oil
Salt and pepper to taste

Wash fennel head and boil in lightly salted water for about twenty minutes. Drain, keeping the water, and wrap fennel in a towel and squeeze out the rest of the water. Chop the fennel and the onion and slice the anchovies thinly. Heat the oil in a skillet and sauté the onions until translucent. Add anchovy fillets, sardines, fennel, and pine nuts and simmer for about ten minutes. Season with salt and pepper.

Prepare pasta in the fennel water according to package directions. Mix with the sauce and heat over low flame for a few minutes to blend the flavors. Serve immediately.

Serves four ○ **Calcium: 45 mg** ○ **Calories per serving: 58**

Basic Components: Calories 58.2; Protein 0.9 g; Carbohydrates 5.7 g; Dietary Fiber 0.12 g; Total–Fat 3.64 g; Saturated Fat 0.56 g; **Vitamins:** Vitamin B6 0.04 mg; Vitamin B12 0 mcg; Vitamin C 14.02 mg; Vitamin D 0 IU; Folate 9.26 mcg; Vitamin K — mcg; **Minerals:** Boron — mcg; Calcium 44.59 mg; Copper 0.02 mg; Magnesium 4.64 mg; Manganese 0.05 mg; Phosphorus 14.2 mg; Sodium 716.92 mg; Zinc 0.05 mg

Potato Gnocchi

THIS IS ANOTHER of those marvelous Italian dishes that sounds more difficult to make than it is. It is delicious as a main course, or as a side dish for fish or meat.

2 lbs boiled potatoes, cooled
2⅓ cups all-purpose flour
2 cups freshly grated Parmesan cheese
1 egg yolk
Dash of salt and pepper
¼ cup unsalted butter
1 clove garlic, crushed
3 tbsp chopped fresh parsley
½ tsp each rosemary, thyme, and dill
1 cup grated Parmesan cheese for garnish

Peel the cooled potatoes and force them through a ricer. Spread them on a smooth surface and mix in the cheese, flour, egg yolk, salt, and pepper. Knead into a soft dough and refrigerate for about an hour. Shape into a roll of dough about as thick as a cigar. If the dough is too soft, add a little more flour. Cut the dough-log into sections about one inch long and flatten them just a little, with a fork. Simmer these gnocchi in lightly salted water for six or seven minutes, drain, and arrange on hot plates. Melt the butter, garlic, and herbs and spoon over the gnocchi and top with the additional grated Parmesan cheese. Serve immediately.

Serves four   ○   **Calcium: 878 mg**   ○   **Calories per serving: 854**

Basic Components: Calories 853.5; Protein 37.35 g; Carbohydrates 104.12 g; Dietary Fiber 6.41 g; Total–Fat 31.7 g; Saturated Fat 19.1 g; **Vitamins:** Vitamin B6 0.74 mg; Vitamin B12 0.97 mcg; Vitamin C 20.95 mg; Vitamin D 30.78 IU; Folate 147.71 mcg; Vitamin K 15.62 mcg; **Minerals:** Boron — mcg; Calcium 877.72 mg; Copper 0.52 mg; Magnesium 94.96 mg; Manganese 0.87 mg; Phosphorus 680.38 mg; Sodium 1,135.25 mg; Zinc 3.23 mg

Fish and Fish Sauces

Baked Bluefish with Cheese and Yogurt

THE CHEESE AND YOGURT add a distinctive flavor to the rich taste of bluefish. The dish is also nice and high in calcium.

¼ cup olive oil
2 medium, thinly sliced zucchini
3 cups seeded, peeled, chopped tomatoes
1 tsp rosemary
1 tsp dill
2 cups farmer cheese
6 tbsp plain, low-fat yogurt
4 bluefish fillets, six to eight oz each

Preheat oven to 400°F.

Heat oil in a skillet and sauté the zucchini for three to four minutes over medium heat. Add tomatoes and spices and continue cooking for two more minutes. Place this mixture in a lightly greased baking dish large enough to hold the fish.

In a bowl combine the cheese and yogurt and coat each fillet with this mixture. Lay the fish on top of the vegetable mixture, spread the rest of the cheese mixture over the top, and bake for twelve to fifteen minutes until fillets are just flaky. Serve at once.

Serves four ○ **Calcium: 925 mg** ○ **Calories per serving: 804**

Basic Components: Calories 804.12; Protein 62.33 g; Carbohydrates 10.29 g; Dietary Fiber 1.74 g; Total–Fat 55.94 g; Saturated Fat 29.47 g; **Vitamins:** Vitamin B6 0.8 mg; Vitamin B12 11.35 mcg; Vitamin C 37.48 mg; Vitamin D 68.04 IU; Folate 25.67 mcg; Vitamin K 6.62 mcg; **Minerals:** Boron — mcg; Calcium 925.08 mg; Copper 0.2 mg; Magnesium 107.88 mg; Manganese 0.2 mg; Phosphorus 1,097.58 mg; Sodium 948.78 mg; Zinc 5.44 mg

Trout Amandine

THIS IS AN EASY-TO-PREPARE, delicious fish dish. It is great in the summer, or anytime year around, for that matter.

    1 egg
    1 cup low-fat milk
    8 trout fillets, about 4 oz each
    ¾ cup all-purpose flour
    ½ cup butter (1 stick)
    ⅔ cup slivered almonds
    3 tbsp fresh lemon juice
    ¼ cup chopped fresh parsley

Preheat oven to 200°F.

Place the almonds in a small skillet over medium heat and sauté (using no oil or shortening) for three to four minutes, until lightly brown. Set aside.

Whisk the egg and milk together in a shallow dish. Dip the fillets in the milk mixture and then dredge them in the flour, shaking off the excess. In a large skillet heat the butter and sauté the fillets for three to four minutes on each side until they are just flaky. Put them on an ovenproof platter and place in the oven to keep them warm.

Add lemon juice and parsley to the small skillet with the almonds and reheat. Place two fillets on each of four warm plates, and spoon the sauce over the fish. Serve at once.

Serves four   ○   **Calcium: 251 mg**   ○   **Calories per serving: 671**

Basic Components: Calories 671.39; Protein 54.05 g; Carbohydrates 12.28 g; Dietary Fiber 2.5 g; Total–Fat 45.05 g; Saturated Fat 18.75 g; **Vitamins:** Vitamin B6 1.46 mg; Vitamin B12 8.75 mcg; Vitamin C 17.12 mg; Vitamin D 30.74 IU; Folate 54.37 mcg; Vitamin K 21.52 mcg; **Minerals:** Boron 0.54 mcg; Calcium 250.67 mg; Copper 0.33 mg; Magnesium 131.68 mg; Manganese 0.56 mg; Phosphorus 781.76 mg; Sodium 107.34 mg; Zinc 1.83 mg

Southern Salmon Cakes

THESE ARE DELICIOUS, easy to make, and perfect for lunch, brunch, or a light supper. They are also loaded with calcium.

    2 cups canned salmon (2 8-oz cans)
    ½ cup whole-grain cracker crumbs
    2 eggs, beaten
    ½ teaspoon dill (or three sprigs chopped fresh dill)
    2 lemons
    1 tbsp olive oil
    Salt and pepper to taste

Drain the salmon well and flake it with a fork. Add the cracker crumbs, two beaten eggs, the strained juice from one of the lemons, and a pinch of salt and pepper to taste. Form these ingredients into cakes and sauté in the olive oil until golden brown. Serve topped with a thin slice of lemon and a sprig of fresh dill or parsley.

Serves six   ○   **Calcium: 209 mg**   ○   **Calories per serving: 195**

Basic Components: Calories 194.93; Protein 18.46 g; Carbohydrates 7.38 g; Dietary Fiber 0.25 g; Total–Fat 9.73 g; Saturated Fat 2.11 g; **Vitamins:** Vitamin B6 0.26 mg; Vitamin B12 0.38 mcg; Vitamin C 3.62 mg; Vitamin D 178.26 IU; Folate 25.15 mcg;

Vitamin K 1.1 mcg; **Minerals:** Boron 0.22 mcg; Calcium 208.88 mg; Copper 0.08 mg; Magnesium 28.01 mg; Manganese 0.1 mg; Phosphorus 286.3 mg; Sodium 502.88 mg; Zinc 1.05 mg

Delicious Fish Sauces

FISH TIP: Many fish, especially those with a strong flavor like tilefish or bluefish, are delicious when topped with a little cheese and mayonnaise and run under the broiler for a few minutes. Blue cheese is particularly good on bluefish—that should be easy to remember.

Mornay Sauce

3 tbsp butter or margarine
3 tbsp all-purpose flour
2 cups low-fat milk
Salt and pepper to taste
¼ cup freshly grated Parmesan cheese
¼ cup grated Swiss cheese

Melt butter and flour in saucepan and stir constantly for three to four minutes. When smooth, remove from heat and add milk while whisking. Return to stove and heat until sauce is thick and creamy. Add cheese and salt and pepper and continue to heat until cheese has melted. This is delicious with any fish. Use two tablespoons of sauce per serving.

Serves ten ○ **Calcium: 106 mg** ○ **Calories per serving: 73**

Basic Components: Calories 73.2; Protein 3.22 g; Carbohydrates 4.04 g; Dietary Fiber 0.06 g; Total–Fat 4.94 g; Saturated Fat 3.09 g; **Vitamins:** Vitamin B6 0.03 mg; Vitamin B12 0.24 mcg; Vitamin C 0.45 mg; Vitamin D 22.3 IU; Folate 6.19 mcg; Vitamin K 1.86 mcg; **Minerals:** Boron 0.69 mcg; Calcium 106.13 mg; Copper 0.01 mg; Magnesium 8.81 mg; Manganese 0.02 mg; Phosphorus 76.93 mg; Sodium 62.41 mg

Orange Sesame Sauce

4 tbsp soy sauce

1½ tbsp sesame oil

1 tsp fresh grated ginger root

4 tbsp rice vinegar

⅔ cup calcium-fortified orange juice

1 tbsp grated orange rind

Whisk all ingredients together. This works well with any kind of fish.

Serves five   ○   **Calcium: 45 mg**   ○   **Calories per serving: 58**

Basic Components: Calories 58.2; Protein 0.9 g; Carbohydrates 5.7 g; Dietary Fiber 0.12 g; Total–Fat 3.64 g; Saturated Fat 0.56 g; **Vitamins:** Vitamin B6 0.04 mg; Vitamin B12 0 mcg; Vitamin C 14.02 mg; Vitamin D 0 IU; Folate 9.26 mcg; Vitamin K — mcg; **Minerals:** Boron — mcg; Calcium 44.59 mg; Copper 0.02 mg; Magnesium 4.64 mg; Manganese 0.05 mg; Phosphorus 14.2 mg; Sodium 71.92 mg; Zinc 0.05 mg

Pesto Sauce

2 cups fresh basil leaves

⅓ cup chopped parsley

2 cloves garlic, peeled

4 walnut halves, shelled

¼ cup pine nuts

½ cup Parmesan cheese, freshly grated

½ cup olive oil

Combine all ingredients in food processor until smooth. Serve at room temperature with most fish. You could also use this with pasta.

Serves five   ○   **Calcium: 139 mg**   ○   **Calories per serving: 268**

Basic Components: Calories 58.2; Protein 0.9 g; Carbohydrates 5.7 g; Dietary Fiber 0.12 g; Fat–Total 3.64 g; Saturated Fat 0.56 g; **Vitamins:** Vitamin B6 0.04 mg; Vitamin B12 0 mcg; Vitamin C 14.02 mg; Vitamin D IU 0 IU; Folate 9.26 mcg; Vitamin K — mcg; **Minerals:** Boron — mcg; Calcium 44.59 mg; Copper 0.02 mg; Magnesium 4.64 mg; Manganese 0.05 mg; Phosphorus 14.2 mg; Sodium 716.92 mg

THE YUMMY HIGH-CALCIUM COOKBOOK FOR KIDS

Plus Tips on Getting More Calcium into Your Child's Diet Every Day

KIDS AND CALCIUM

OUR KIDS ARE IN CRISIS. Seventy percent of girls between six and eleven don't get enough calcium in their diets. Sixty percent of boys in the same age group are calcium deficient. And it gets worse. During their teenage years (twelve through nineteen), 86% of teenage girls do not get the minimum Recommended Daily Allowance of calcium (1,200 mg per day, for this age group). This is particularly troubling, since it is during the growth spurt between the ages of ten and thirteen that girls develop 15% of their adult height, 50% of their adult weight, and 45% of their bone structure.

The other major health problem for kids today is obesity. Twenty-five percent of American children are seriously overweight. In fact, the percentage of obese children between six and eleven has doubled since 1980, from 7 to 15%. The increase was even greater in twelve- to nineteen-year-olds (from 5 to 15% in the same time period), and a shocking 10.2% of preschool children are seriously overweight, according to the National Center for Health Statistics.

If a child is overweight at age four, he or she has a 20% chance of carrying that weight into adulthood. If a child is overweight as an adolescent, he or she has an 80% chance of becoming an overweight adult. What's more, obesity in children greatly increases their risk of developing Type 2 diabetes, hypertension, cholesterol problems, and asthma, as well as depression and other psychological disorders.

There is a way to solve both problems. It all depends on adjusting a child's diet and keeping him or her active. Lack of exercise, as well as poor diet, is a cause of weakened bones and obesity in children, so do everything you can to make sure your child gets plenty of exercise. In addition, if you are careful to see that your children eat a balanced diet rich in calcium and low in fat (and the empty calories that come from sugar), there is no question that you will be helping them have happier, healthier, longer lives.

Easier said than done, of course, but here are some simple ways to get started:

○ Make sure your child drinks one eight-ounce glass of low-fat milk a day. Up until the age of two, children need whole milk, but after age two, low-fat is the answer. This will ensure at least 300 mg of calcium per day.

○ Have your child drink one eight-ounce glass of calcium-fortified orange juice or grapefruit juice every day. This will give him or her an additional 350 to 400 mg of calcium.

○ Make plain, low-fat yogurt into a tempting daily snack by dressing it up with fresh berries and nuts.

○ Encourage calcium-fortified cereal at breakfast, and have your kids drink the milk that is left in the bowl.

○ Try to limit soft drinks to one a day.

Just following these five simple steps could add as much as 1,000 mg of calcium to your child's diet each day, and it could also be the first step toward helping your children develop healthy eating habits.

QUICK, HIGH-CALCIUM FOODS THAT KIDS LOVE

1. **Tuna Melt:** Prepare tuna salad with low-fat mayonnaise and chopped celery, spread it on whole-grain bread, top it with a slice of Swiss, American, or cheddar cheese, and run it under the broiler, or place in a toaster oven for eight to ten minutes until the cheese has melted completely and turned slightly brown. You could make this with canned salmon salad as well.

2. **Cheese Dogs:** Slice pure beef or turkey hot dogs lengthwise, two thirds of the way through. Spread open and top with sliced or grated cheddar or American cheese. Place under the broiler or in a toaster oven until the hot dog has heated through and the cheese has browned.

3. **Grilled Cheese and Tomato Sandwiches:** Lightly butter both sides of two slices of whole-grain bread. Place two slices of Swiss, cheddar, or American cheese on one slice and tomatoes on the other. Place slices together and sauté in a skillet for about three minutes on each side, until the cheese has melted and the bread has turned a crunchy, golden brown.

4. **Veggie Melt:** Combine a variety of fresh, peeled vegetables (zucchini; tomatoes; squash; unpeeled red, orange, or green peppers; onions; steamed broccoli; or cauliflower, for example) on a slice of whole-grain bread. Top with two slices of Swiss, cheddar, or American cheese and place under broiler or in toaster oven until vegetables are hot and cheese has melted completely.

5. **Tasty Tacos:** Combine chopped vegetables (as above) with two ounces chopped cheddar, Swiss, or American cheese. Stuff filling into pre-prepared taco shells, and heat according to package directions. Top with additional grated cheese before serving.

6. **Mini Pizza:** Break a whole-grain English muffin into two halves and top with salsa and Swiss, cheddar, or American cheese. Bake in a 375°F oven for ten to twenty minutes or pop into a toaster oven. The pizza will be ready when the cheese has melted completely and turned a golden brown.

7. **Frozen Yogurt Parfait:** In a glass bowl or parfait glass, place two scoops of low-fat, vanilla frozen yogurt and top with banana slices and chopped nuts. Add one tablespoon of chocolate syrup for a special treat.

8. **Fluffy Hot Chocolate:** Heat one cup low-fat milk or calcium-fortified soy milk in a small saucepan until bubbles start to appear. Remove from heat and stir in two tablespoons cocoa mix and one tablespoon maple syrup. Beat until smooth and frothy with a wire whisk. Top with a dollop of whipped heavy cream and a sprig of fresh mint.

9. **Scrumptious Scrambled Eggs:** In a small mixing bowl, whisk two eggs and a quarter cup low-fat milk with two tablespoons grated Parmesan or cheddar cheese. Add one teaspoon butter to a small skillet and scramble eggs. Top with fresh parsley.

10. **Special PB and J:** Add five or six finely chopped fresh figs to half a cup of peanut butter. Using whole-grain bread, make your child's favorite peanut butter and jelly sandwich, using this special high-calcium peanut butter.

HIGH-CALCIUM RECIPES FOR KIDS

Four Fabulous Smoothies

These divine drinks can be made ahead of time and stored in the refrigerator. You can use them as snacks or enjoy them at breakfast. Kids love them, too.

Apricot Ambrosia
Fresh Fruit Frosty
Peanut Butter Delight
Strawberry-Banana Surprise

Lunch or Dinner

These recipes are favorites of adults, too.

The Famous French Croque Monsieur Sandwich
Macaroni and Cheese

Snacks

These are great for adults as well as children.

Crunchy Cheese Crackers
Good Old-Fashioned Cheese Straws
Old-Fashioned Pimento Cheese Spread

Dessert

Kids love this, but it is also a great dessert for any grown-up spring or summer meal.

Beautiful Butterscotch Pudding

Four Fabulous Smoothies

Apricot Ambrosia

1½ cups canned apricots, drained

½ cup plain, low-fat yogurt

½ cup skim milk

3 tbsp nonfat dry milk

3 tbsp low-fat sour cream

1 tbsp sugar

1 lemon (juice, strained)

Combine all ingredients in a blender or food processor and blend until smooth. Serve immediately or store in a covered glass container in the refrigerator. Makes 24 ounces.

Calcium: 682 mg ◯ **Calories: 476**

Basic Components: Calories 475.5; Protein 20.3 g; Carbohydrates 86.2 g; Dietary Fiber 6.09 g; Total–Fat 7.85 g; Saturated Fat 4.91 g; **Vitamins:** Vitamin B6 0.39 mg; Vitamin B12 1.71 mcg; Vitamin C 44.66 mg; Vitamin D 50.95 IU; Folate 39.42 mcg; Vitamin K 0.39 mcg; **Minerals:** Boron 1.84 mcg; Calcium 682.42 mg; Copper 0.25 mg; Magnesium 94.43 mg; Manganese 0.2 mg; Phosphorus 569.45 mg; Sodium 268.82 mg; Zinc 2.56 mg

Fresh Fruit Frosty

1 cup honeydew melon

½ cup plain, low-fat yogurt

½ cup skim milk

3 tbsp nonfat dry milk

½ cup fresh strawberries or raspberries

½ tsp vanilla extract

½ tsp sugar

Combine all ingredients in a blender or food processor and blend until frothy. Serve at once or store in a covered glass container in the refrigerator. Makes 18 ounces.

Calcium: 583 mg ○ **Calories: 207**

Basic Components: Calories 270.17; Protein 17.04 g; Carbohydrates 45.9 g; Dietary Fiber 2.97 g; Total–Fat 2.6 g; Saturated Fat 1.43 g; **Vitamins:** Vitamin B6 0.33 mg; Vitamin B12 1.71 mcg; Vitamin C 95.55 mg; Vitamin D 50.95 IU; Folate 51.55 mcg; Vitamin K 1.64 mcg; **Minerals:** Boron 1.84 mcg; Calcium 582.72 mg; Copper 0.15 mg; Magnesium 75.96 mg; Manganese 0.29 mg; Phosphorus 475.67 mg; Sodium 244.9 mg; Zinc 2.36 mg

Peanut Butter Delight

½ cup skim milk
2 tbsp nonfat dry milk
2 tbsp peanut butter
4 ice cubes
1 banana, sliced
1 tsp sugar
Dash of cinnamon

Combine all ingredients in a blender or food processor and purée. Serve immediately or store in a covered glass container in the refrigerator. Makes 10 ounces.

Calcium: 319 mg ○ **Calories: 398**

Basic Components: Calories 397.52; Protein 17.56 g; Carbohydrates 49.42 g; Dietary Fiber 4.72 g; Total–Fat 17.2 g; Saturated Fat 3.73 g; **Vitamins:** Vitamin B6 0.93 mg; Vitamin B12 0.9 mcg; Vitamin C 13.68 mg; Vitamin D 49.2 IU; Folate 57.74 mcg; Vitamin K 3.79 mcg; **Minerals:** Boron 1.85 mcg; Calcium 318.75 mg; Copper 0.18 mg; Magnesium 118.59 mg; Manganese 0.33 mg; Phosphorus 374.13 mg; Sodium 274.37 mg; Zinc 2.04 mg

Strawberry-Banana Surprise

1 cup fresh sliced strawberries
1 cup sliced banana
½ cup plain, low-fat yogurt
½ cup skim milk
3 tbsp nonfat dry milk
3 tbsp low-fat sour cream
Juice of one lemon, strained

Combine all ingredients in a blender or food processor and blend until smooth. Serve at once or store in the refrigerator in a covered glass container. Makes 24 ounces.

Calcium: 671 mg   ◯   **Calories: 439**

Basic Components: Calories 439.24; Protein 20.55 g; Carbohydrates 75.35 g; Dietary Fiber 7.65 g; Total–Fat 9.03 g; Saturated Fat 5.21 g; **Vitamins:** Vitamin B6 1.16 mg; Vitamin B12 1.71 mcg; Vitamin C 134.5 mg; Vitamin D 50.95 IU; Folate 90.48 mcg; Vitamin K 3.63 mcg; **Minerals:** Boron 1.84 mcg; Calcium 670.61 mg; Copper 0.28 mg; Magnesium 117.93 mg; Manganese 0.72 mg; Phosphorus 557.54 mg; Sodium 257.22 mg; Zinc 2.61 mg

Lunch or Dinner

The Famous French
Croque Monsieur Sandwich

THIS MAKES A FABULOUS BRUNCH or luncheon dish. It is sophisticated, easy to make, delicious, and high in calcium.

2 slices 12-grain bread, crusts removed
2 ⅛-inch slices Gruyère or Swiss cheese
1 ⅛-inch slice baked ham

Dijon mustard
2 tbsp butter or margarine
Fresh parsley, dill, or cilantro

Spread mustard on each slice of bread. Then place the sliced cheese on each slice and the ham on one of the slices. Put the slices together and trim off excess cheese and ham. Heat the butter or margarine in a skillet. Brush the top of the sandwich with the melted butter or margarine. Place the sandwich, unbuttered side down, in the skillet and brown slowly. Turn it over and brown the other side. Put the skillet in a 350°F oven and heat until cheese is completely melted. Place on a plate, garnish with a sprig of parsley, dill, or cilantro and serve at once.

Serves one   ○   Calcium: 692 mg   ○   Calories: 602

Basic Components: Calories 602.07; Protein 27.83 g; Carbohydrates 24.62 g; Dietary Fiber 3.33 g; Total–Fat 44.43 g; Saturated Fat 25.74 g; **Vitamins:** Vitamin B6 0.35 mg; Vitamin B12 1.19 mcg; Vitamin C 0.16 mg; Vitamin D 21.27 IU; Folate 49.24 mcg; Vitamin K — mcg; **Minerals:** Boron — mcg; Calcium 629.26 mg; Copper 0.17 mg; Magnesium 53.35 mg; Manganese 0.79 mg; Phosphorus 502.8 mg; Sodium 851.95 mg; Zinc 3.43 mg

Macaroni and Cheese

MOST KIDS ADORE MACARONI AND CHEESE, but I've never known an adult who didn't love it, too. There are many variations on this recipe, but this one is especially delicious.

3 oz provolone cheese
3 oz Fontina cheese
3 oz sharp cheddar cheese
½ cup low-fat milk
1 lb macaroni
¼ cup butter
½ cup freshly grated Parmesan cheese
⅓ cup chopped parsley

Grate the first three cheeses into a bowl. Heat the milk just to boiling and pour over the cheeses. Let this mixture stand for about half an hour. Meanwhile, bring lightly salted water to a boil and cook the macaroni for ten to twelve minutes until just tender, and drain well. Melt the butter in a large, deep pan and toss the macaroni in the melted butter. Pour in the milk and cheese mixture and add the Parmesan cheese, and heat until the cheese melts. Serve immediately topped with the chopped parsley.

Serves four   ○   **Calcium: 623 mg**   ○   **Calories: 790**

Basic Components: Calories 789.62; Protein 34.43 g; Carbohydrates 81.6 g; Dietary Fiber 3.76 g; Total–Fat 35.63 g; Saturated Fat 21.47 g; **Vitamins:** Vitamin B6 0.17 mg; Vitamin B12 1.11 mcg; Vitamin C 6.95 mg; Vitamin D 29.14 IU; Folate 36.97 mcg; Vitamin K 29 mcg; **Minerals:** Boron 0.46 mcg; Calcium 623.43 mg; Copper 0.31 mg; Magnesium 76.78 mg; Manganese 0.81 mg; Phosphorus 546.27 mg; Sodium 680.51 mg; Zinc 4.06 mg

Snacks

Crunchy Cheese Crackers

THESE CALCIUM-RICH CRACKERS are great snacks for kids, and you can also serve them at cocktail parties.

> 1 lb sharp cheddar cheese
> 8 tbsp butter
> 2 cups flour
> Dash of salt and pepper
> ½ tsp Tabasco sauce

Preheat the oven to 325°F.

Grate the cheese. Blend it with the chopped butter in a food processor or electric mixer. Sift in two cups flour, salt, pepper, and a dash of Tabasco. Mix well. Chill the dough for an hour and a half. Make it into small balls and roll them out into thin, cookie-shaped rounds. Place in the oven on a lightly greased cookie sheet and bake for about thirty minutes, until they are lightly brown on the bottom but not on the top. Let cool and store in your cookie jar.

Makes about eighty crackers   ○   **Calcium: 122 mg**   ○   **Calories: 130**

Basic Components: Calories 129.89; Protein 5.13 g; Carbohydrates 7.21 g; Dietary Fiber 0.25 g; Total–Fat 8.94 g; Saturated Fat 5.6 g; **Vitamins:** Vitamin B6 0.02 mg; Vitamin B12 0.14 mcg; Vitamin C 0 mg; Vitamin D 4.3 IU; Folate 17.24 mcg; Vitamin K 0.55 mcg; **Minerals:** Boron — mcg; Calcium 122.32 mg; Copper 0.02 mg; Magnesium 6.77 mg; Manganese 0.06 mg; Phosphorus 96.05 mg; Sodium 104.49 mg; Zinc 0.58 mg

Good Old-Fashioned Cheese Straws

YOU CAN BAKE THESE AHEAD OF TIME and then freeze them until you have a party, or just munch on them at snack time (with the kids, of course).

  1 cup all-purpose flour
  1 cup grated sharp cheddar cheese
  Salt and pepper to taste
  ¼ cup butter
  1 egg, beaten

Preheat the oven to 425°F. Mix together flour, cheese, salt, and pepper. Cut in the butter until the mixture looks like corn meal. Stir in the beaten egg, and knead dough until it forms a ball. Add a little water if necessary. Roll the dough thin on a lightly floured board and cut into two-and-a-half-inch strips. Place the strips on a greased cookie sheet and bake six to eight minutes, until lightly browned.

Makes about eighteen cheese straws   ○   **48 mg (per straw)**   ○
Calories: 77

Basic Components: Calories 77.02; Protein 2.65 g; Carbohydrates 5.42 g; Dietary Fiber 0.19 g; Total–Fat 4.95 g; Saturated Fat 2.99 g; **Vitamins:** Vitamin B6 0.01 mg; Vitamin B12 0.08 mcg; Vitamin C 0 mg; Vitamin D 3.94 IU; Folate 13.22 mcg;

Vitamin K 0.23 mcg; **Minerals:** Boron 0.04 mcg; Calcium 48.41 mg; Copper 0.01 mg; Magnesium 3.63 mg; Manganese 0.05 mg; Phosphorus 45.3 mg; Sodium 42.97 mg; Zinc 0.28 mg

Old-Fashioned Pimento Cheese Spread

MAKE THIS AHEAD OF TIME and keep refrigerated until ready to serve on dark, whole-grain bread, or as an appetizer on celery.

> 12 oz grated cheddar cheese
> 2 4-oz jars drained pimentos
> 1 cup low-fat mayonnaise

After draining the pimentos, put all the ingredients into a blender or food processor and blend until smooth. Store in glass container in the refrigerator.

Makes three cups ○ **Calcium: 92 mg (per tbsp)** ○
Calories: 83

Basic Components: Calories 82.71; Protein 3.3 g; Carbohydrates 1.35 g; Dietary Fiber 0.17 g; Total–Fat 7.15 g; Saturated Fat 3.12 g; **Vitamins:** Vitamin B6 0.03 mg; Vitamin B12 0.1 mcg; Vitamin C 7.18 mg; Vitamin D 1.52 IU; Folate 2.78 mcg; Vitamin K 0.38 mcg; **Minerals:** Boron — mcg; Calcium 92.22 mg; Copper 0.01 mg; Magnesium 4.05 mg; Manganese 0.01 mg; Phosphorus 71.36 mg; Sodium 150.83 mg; Zinc 0.41 mg

Dessert

Beautiful Butterscotch Pudding

YOU CAN TOP THIS DELICIOUS DESSERT off with a little additional whipped cream if you want to be truly indulgent.

2 cups low-fat milk
1 tbsp butter
4 tbsp light-brown sugar
1 tsp vanilla extract
Pinch of salt
4 tbsp cornstarch

Combine milk, butter, and three tablespoons of the sugar, vanilla, and salt in a saucepan and heat until hot, but do not let it boil. Put the cornstarch in a separate bowl. Pour in half the milk mixture and whisk briskly, then return it to the saucepan with remaining milk mixture and return the pan to the heat. Simmer, stirring constantly until it becomes thick and shiny, about five minutes. Put the mixture in a serving bowl, sprinkle the top with the remaining brown sugar, cover the bowl tightly with plastic wrap, and refrigerate until cool.

Serves four ○ **Calcium: 163 mg** ○ **Calories: 161**

Basic Components: Calories 161.47; Protein 4.06 g; Carbohydrates 26.65 g; Dietary Fiber 0.07 g; Total–Fat 4.14 g; Saturated Fat 2.57 g; **Vitamins:** Vitamin B6 0.06 mg; Vitamin B12 0.45 mcg; Vitamin C 1.18 mg; Vitamin D 50.76 IU; Folate 6.46 mcg; Vitamin K 4.88 mcg; **Minerals:** Boron 1.83 mcg; Calcium 162.87 mg; Copper 0.06 mg; Magnesium 21.29 mg; Manganese 0.05 mg; Phosphorus 122.3 mg; Sodium 68.17 mg; Zinc 0.51 mg

RESOURCES

Osteoporosis Organizations, Internet Sites,
Food-Labeling Information,
and Support Groups

IF YOU NEED HELP or advice about osteoporosis or related illnesses, there are many fine organizations ready and willing to direct you to the resources you need.

Osteoporosis

American Academy of Orthopedic Surgeons
6300 North River Road
Rosemont, Illinois 60018
847-823-7186
www.aaos.org

American Society for Bone and Mineral Research
2025 M Street, N.W., Suite 800
Washington, D.C. 20036
202-367-1161
www.asbmr.org

Foundation for Osteoporosis Research
300 27th Street, Suite 103
Oakland, California 94612
888-266-3015
www.fore.org

International Society for Clinical Densitometry
This organization has seven regional representatives but no central mailing address, so check the website to find the e-mail address for the representative from your region.
E-mail: *ascd@dc.sba.com*
www.iscd.org

National Osteoporosis Foundation
1232 22nd Street, N.W.
Washington, D.C. 20037-1292
202-223-2226
800-223-9994
www.nof.org

National Osteoporosis and Related Bone Diseases
National Resource Center
1232 22nd Street, N.W.
Washington, D.C. 20037-1292
800-624-2663
www.osteo.org

Osteoporosis Society of Canada
33 Laird Drive
Toronto, ON M4G 3S9
416-696-2663
www.osteoporosis.ca

Osteoporosis Links
www.pslgroup.com/Osteoporosis

Women's Health

American College of Obstetricians and Gynecologists
409 12th Street, S.W.
Washington, D.C. 20024
202-638-5577
www.acog.org

The Hormone Foundation
4350 East-West Highway, Suite 500
Bethesda, Maryland 20814
800-HORMONE (800-467-6663)
www.hormone.org

The Jacobs Institute of Women's Health
409 12th Street, S.W.
Washington, D.C. 20024
202-863-4990
www.jiwh.org

National Association of Nurse Practitioners in Women's Health
503 Capital Court N.E., Suite 300

Washington, D.C. 20002
202-543-9693
www.npwh.org

National Women's Health Network
514 10th Street, N.W., Suite 400
Washington, D.C. 20004
202-347-1140
www.womenshealthnetwork.org

National Women's Health Resource Center
157 Broad Street, Suite 315
Red Bank, New Jersey 07701
877-986-9472 (toll free)
www.healthywomen.org

North American Menopause Society
P.O. Box 94527
Cleveland, OH 44101
440-442-7550
800-774-5342
www.menopause.org

The Society of Obstetricians and Gynecologists of Canada
780 Echo Drive
Ottawa, ON K1S 5R7
613-730-4192
800-561-2416 (toll free in Canada only)
www.sogc.org

SOURCES

*for Help and Information
on Related Conditions*

Aging

American Association of Retired Persons
601 East Street, N.W.
Washington, D.C. 20029
202-434-2277
www.aarp.org

American Geriatrics Society Foundation for Health in Aging (FHA)
350 Fifth Avenue, Suite 801
New York, New York 10018
212-755-6810
www.healthinaging.org

National Association of Area Agencies on Aging
1112 16th Street, N.W.
Washington, D.C. 20036
202-296-8130
www.n4a.org

National Council on the Aging
409 Third Street, S.W., Suite 200
Washington, D.C. 20024
www.ncoa.org

National Institute on Aging
Public Information Office, Room 5C27
31 Center Drive, MSC 2292
Bethesda, Maryland 20892
301-496-1752

800-222-2225
www.nia.nih.gov

Older Women's League
1750 New York Avenue, N.W., Suite 350
Washington, D.C.
202-783-6686
www.owl-national.org

Alcohol

Alcoholics Anonymous
P.O. Box 459
Grand Central Station
New York, New York 10163
212-870-3400
www.aa.org

National Council on Alcoholism and Drug Dependence
12 West 21st Street
New York, New York 10010
212-206-6770
800-NCA-CALL (800-622-2255)
www.ncadd.org

Alzheimer's Disease

Alzheimer's Association
919 North Michigan Avenue, Suite 1100
Chicago, Illinois 60611-1676
800-272-3900
www.alz.org

Alzheimer's Disease Education and Referral Center
P.O. Box 8250
Silver Spring, Maryland 20907-8250
301-495-3311
800-483-4380
www.alzheimers.org

Arthritis

The Arthritis Foundation
National Office
1330 West Peachtree Street, Suite 100

Atlanta, Georgia 30309
404-872-7100
800-283-7800
www.arthritis.org

National Institute of Arthritis and Musculoskeletal and Skin Diseases

National Institutes of Health
Building 31, Room 4C02
31 Center Drive, MSC 2350
Bethesda, Maryland 20892-2350
301-496-8190
www.niams.nih.gov

General Medicine

American Medical Association

515 North State Street
Chicago, Illinois 60610
312-464-5000
www.ama-assn.org

National Council on Patient Information and Education

4915 St. Elmo Avenue, Suite 505
Bethesda, Maryland 20814-6053
301-656-8565
www.talkaboutrx.org

National Institutes of Health

9000 Rockville Pike
Bethesda, Maryland 20892
301-496-4000
www.nih.gov

U.S. Department of Health and Human Services

200 Independence Avenue, S.W.
Washington, D.C. 20201
202-619-0257
www.os.dhhs.gov

U.S. Food and Drug Administration

5600 Fishers Lane
Rockville, Maryland 20857-0001
888-463-6332
www.fda.gov

Heart Problems

American Heart Association
7272 Greenville Avenue
Dallas, Texas 75231
214-373-6300
www.americanheart.org

Mental Health

National Mental Health Association
1021 Prince Street
Alexandria, Virginia 22314-2971
703-684-7722
800-969-NMHA (800-969-6642)
www.nmha.org

National Eating Disorders Association
603 Stewart Street, Suite 803
Seattle, Washington 98101
800-931-2237
206-382-3587
www.nationaleatingdisorders.org

Pain Relief

American Chronic Pain Association
P.O. Box 850
Rocklin, California 95677
916-632-0922
www.theacpa.org

Rehabilitation

National Rehabilitation Information Center
1010 Wayne Avenue, Suite 800
Silver Spring, Maryland 20910
800-346-2742
www.naric.com

Sleep Problems

National Sleep Foundation
1522 K Street, N.W., Suite 500
Washington, D.C. 20005
202-374-3471
www.sleepfoundation.org

Smoking

American Lung Association
61 Broadway
New York, New York 10006
212-315-8700
800-586-4872
www.lungusa.org

Stroke and Nerve Damage

National Institute of Neurological Disorders and Stroke
P.O. Box 5801
Bethesda, Maryland 20824
301-496-5751
800-352-9424
www.ninds.nih.gov

National Stroke Association
9707 E. Easter Lane
Englewood, Colorado 80112
800-STROKES (800-787-6537)
www.stroke.org

Thyroid Problems

Thyroid Foundation of America
410 Stuart Street
Boston, Massachusetts 02116
800-832-8321
www.tsh.org

Urinary Problems

National Association for Continence
P.O. Box 1019
Charleston, South Carolina 29402-1019
864-579-7900
800-BLADDER (800-252-3337)
www.nafc.org

Whole-Food Resources

Atkins Center
152 East 55th Street
New York, New York 10022
212-758-2110
www.atkins.com

Bob's Red Mill National Foods
5209 Southeast International Way
Milwaukee, Oregon 97222
800-349-2173
www.bobsredmill.com

ECO Directory Greenleaf Media
2501 University Avenue
Madison, Wisconsin 53705
608-233-1737
www.naturalfoodsdirectory.com

Ener-G Foods
5960 First Avenue South
P.O. Box 84487
Seattle, Washington 98124-5787
800-331-5222
www.ener-g.com

New Earth Natural Foods
1605 State Road
Cuyahoga Falls, Ohio 44223-1303
330-929-2415
www.newearthnaturalfoods.com

Wild Oats Natural Marketplace
Wild Oats Markets, Inc.
3375 Mitchell Lane
Boulder, Colorado 80301
303-440-5220
www.wildoats.com

To find out how much calcium and other nutrients are in the foods you eat, you can check *www.foodingridientsfirst.com*.

Or you can refer to individual manufacturers' websites, including:

www.cocacola.com
www.generalmills.com
www.kraft.com
www.minutemaid.com
www.pepsi.com
www.tropicana.com

For other companies, simply refer to the label on the package for the name of the manufacturer and their website address.

GLOSSARY

ABSORPTIOMETRY: A medical test to measure bone density.

ACTIVELLA™: The brand name for a combined continuous hormone replacement preparation that contains 1 mg of estradiol and 0.5 mg of norethindrone. It is FDA approved for the prevention of osteoporosis and is marketed by Upjohn Pharmaceuticals and Pharmacia.

ACTONEL™: The brand name for risedronate sodium, manufactured by Procter & Gamble Pharmaceuticals. This bisphosphonate is FDA approved for the prevention of osteoporosis at a dose of 5 mg per day. It is an oral medication and is available by prescription only.

AEROBIC EXERCISE: Rhythmic, continuous body movement that uses the large muscles of the body for five minutes or more, using oxygen as fuel. Aerobic literally means "with oxygen."

AGILITY: Ability of the body to move quickly and easily while maintaining balance and control.

AGONIST: A drug that acts like a natural hormone or compound. An estrogen agonist would produce an effect similar to estrogen, for example.

ALENDRONATE: The chemical name for the bisphosphonate Fosamax™, a nonhormonal medication that has been approved by the FDA for the prevention and treatment of osteoporosis in postmenopausal women. It is made by Merck & Co.

ALPHA BLOCKERS: Drugs that help relax blood vessels so blood can more easily flow through the arteries. They may help lower blood pressure and symptoms caused by enlarged prostate. They include Cardura™ (doxazosin), Flomax™ (tamsulosin), Hytrin™ (terazosin), and Minipress™ (prazosin).

AMENORRHEA: The absence of menstrual periods in premenopausal women.

ANAEROBIC: Without oxygen.

ANAEROBIC EXERCISE: This type of exercise allows muscles to work temporarily without oxygen, replenishing oxygen at a later time. Strength training with weights and elastic bands is a good anaerobic exercise that can build bone and increase the speed of the body's metabolism.

ANALGESICS: Medications to help relieve pain. They include **acetaminophen** (Anacin™, Genapap™, Panadol™, Panex™, and Tylenol™); **aspirin** (Arthritis Pain Formula, Asciptin™, Bufferin™, Ecotrin™, Empirin™, Halfprin™, ZORprin™, and others); **aspirin-like medications** (Disalcid [Doan's™, Magan™, Mobidin™, and others], Dolobid™, Trilisate™, and others); **medications containing aspirin** (Darvon Compound, Talwin Compound, and others); **narcotic pain relievers** (Darvon™, Demerol™, Dilaudia™, Duragesic™, Hycodan™, Levo-Dromoran™, OxyContin™, Stadol™, Talwin™, codeine, and others.

ANDROGENS: A group of hormones related to the male sex hormone testosterone, androsterone, and dehydroepinadrosterone (DHEA).

ANEMIA: A condition in which you do not have enough red blood cells, caused by blood loss, decrease in the production of red blood cells, or an increase in red blood cell destruction. Fatigue is a symptom of this condition.

ANOREXIA NERVOSA: An eating disorder that usually affects but is not limited to young women with a poor body self-image, which leads to an exaggerated fear of being fat. They almost starve themselves to avoid gaining weight, and this can lead to osteoporosis and other diseases, as well as premature death.

ANTACID: Medication that decreases the amount of acid in the stomach by neutralizing stomach acid. Antacids contain aluminum, calcium, magnesium, or sodium bicarbonate. They include **those containing aluminum**: Alamag™, AlternaGEL™, Amphojel™, Basaljel™, Di-Gel™, Gaviscon™, Maalox™, Riopan™, and others; **those containing calcium**: Alka-mints™, Alkerts™, Amitone™, Chooz™, Discarbosil™, Equilet™, Mallamint™, Rolaids™, Titralic Plus™, Titralac™, Tums™, and others; **those containing magnesium**: Alamag™, Alkerts™, Di-Gel™, Maalox™, Phillips' Milk of Magnesia™, Mylanta™, Rolaids™, and others; and **those containing sodium bicarbonate**: Bellans™, Bromo-Seltzer™, Citrocarbonate™, Gaviscon™, and others.

ANTIBIOTICS: Medications that help destroy bacteria or keep bacteria from growing. They include sulfa drugs, amoxicillin, erythromycin, minocycline, and penicillin, under many different trade names. When used for a prolonged period of time they can interfere with calcium absorption.

ANTICOAGULANT: Blood-thinning medication that helps prevent new blood clots from forming and existing clots from getting bigger. Coumadin™ (warfarin), heparin, and Levenox™ (enoxaparin) are among them.

ANTIDEPRESSANTS: Medications to prevent or relieve the symptoms of depression. They include: **MAO** (monoamine oxidase) **inhibitors** (Marplan™, Nardil™, Parnate™, and others); **selective serotonin reuptake inhibitors** (**SSRIs**) (Clexa™, Luvooox™, Paxil™, and Zoloft)™; **tricyclic antidepressants** (Anafranil™, Asendion, Elavil, Norpramine, Parnclor, Sinequan, Surmontil, Tofranil, and Vivactil); **others** (Desyrel, Ludiomil, Remeron, Serzone, Wellbutrin, and others).

ANTIHISTAMINES: Medications that help block the effects of histamine, a natural substance that makes the nose stuffy and eyes watery. Some make you sleepy and relieve the symptoms of anxiety or sleeplessness. They include **non-drowsy** Allegra™, Claritin™, Hismanal™, Seldane™, Zyrtec™, and others. Those that **cause drowsiness** include: Atarax™, Benadryl™, Excedrin P.M.™, Nytol™, Sleep-Eze 3™, Sominex™, Tavist™, Tylenol P.M.™, Unisom™, Vistaril™, and others.

ANTI-INFLAMMATORY: Medication to help reduce the symptoms of inflammation such as swelling, redness, and pain.

ANTIRESORPTIVE DRUGS: These medications decrease the activity of the osteoclasts (bone clearers), and so decrease the breakdown of bone.

ARRHYTHMIA: Irregular (fast, slow, or abnormal) heartbeat.

ARTERIOSCLEROSIS: Hardening of the arteries.

ARTERY: A blood vessel that carries blood from the heart to other parts of the body. Veins provide the passageway for the blood coming back to the heart.

ARTHRITIS: An inflammation of the joints that may cause pain, swelling, and redness. In severe cases, the joint may be destroyed.

ATHEROSCLEROSIS: Hardening of the arteries, often caused by too much cholesterol inside the arteries, which leads to heart disease.

ATROPIC: A term to describe the condition of deterioration.

ATROPIC VAGINITIS: A thinning of the vaginal tissue caused by estrogen deficiency. It can lead to infections, dryness, and painful intercourse.

BARBITURATE: An addictive medication that can help sleep and produce a calming effect like sedation. These drugs include: Alurate™, Amytal™, Butisol™, Luminal™, Mebaral™, Nembutal™, Seconal™, and others.

BETA BLOCKERS: Medications to help slow down the heart beat, decrease the heart's need for oxygen, and lower blood pressure. They include: Betagan™, Betapace™, Coreg™, Cosopi™, Interal™, Lavatol™, Normodyne™, Tenormin™, Zebeta™, Ziac™, and others.

BICONCAVE FRACTURE: A type of spinal fracture in which the back and front of the vertebrae remain intact but the upper and lower central part of the vertebrae collapse.

BIOTIN: One of the B-complex vitamins. It is essential for many of our enzyme systems and is found in abundance in egg yolk, milk, liver, and yeast.

BISPHOSPHONATES: A medication that decreases the osteoclast activity that in turn decreases bone breakdown. These drugs are especially effective in increasing bone density in your spine and hips. Fosamax™ (alendronate) is a bisphosphonate, FDA approved for both men and women. It may be particularly effective if your osteoporosis is caused by steroid use. It may reduce your risk of fracture by 50%. Actonel (risedronate) is effective for women but has not been approved for men.

BMD: The acronym for bone mineral density.

BODY MASS INDEX (BMI): The ratio of weight in kilograms to height in meters. This is used to assess body weight. A BMI anywhere between 19 and 25 is considered healthy.

BONE DENSITOMETRY: The measurement of bone density or strength.

BONE DENSITY: The amount of mineral in any given volume of bone, giving it its strength and thickness.

BONE MASS: The total amount of bone mineral in the body. Bone mass is different from bone density, but the terms are often used interchangeably.

BONE REMODELING: The cycle of bone growth, maintenance, and repair in which old bone is dissolved by osteoclasts and new bone is created by osteoblasts.

BULIMIA: An eating disorder in which a person binges on food and then makes herself or himself vomit in an effort to stay thin. See *anorexia nervosa.*

BURSITIS: The inflammation of bursa, which is a small sac (tissue space) filled with fluid to make movement easier. Located in the knee and elbow, among other places.

CALCIMAR™: The trade name for salmon calcitonin, an FDA-approved injection for the treatment of osteoporosis in postmenopausal women. It is manufactured by Rhone-Poulene Rorer.

CALCITONIN: A peptide hormone made in the thyroid gland that lowers the amount of calcium in the blood. In humans it acts to decrease the formation and absorptive activity of osteoclasts (bone clearers). It helps regulate the amount of calcium in the blood, and may decrease spine fractures by 40%. It is taken as a nasal spray and causes nasal irritation in about 12% of users.

CALCIUM: The most important mineral in your body. It is essential to the development and maintenance of a healthy skeleton. If your calcium intake is inadequate, the body takes calcium from your skeleton to keep the calcium blood levels normal. It is also essential for healthy muscle contraction, transmission of nerve impulses, cell function, and blood clotting.

CALCIUM CARBONATE: A naturally occurring form of calcium often used in supplements. It is more difficult to absorb than calcium citrate.

CALCIUM CITRATE, CALCIUM GLUTONATE, AND CALCIUM LACTATE: These are synthetic forms of calcium often used in supplements. Citrate is the easiest to absorb.

CALCIUM SUPPLEMENTS: These medications help increase the amount of calcium in the body. They include: Calcet Plus™ (calcium carbonate), Caltrate™ (calcium/vitamin D), Citracal™ (calcium citrate), New-Calglucon™ (calcium gluconate), Os-Cal 500™ (calcium carbonate), Posture™ (calcium phosphate), Viacin™ (calcium carbonate/vitamins D and K), and others.

CARBOHYDRATE: A substance found primarily in starchy and sugary foods such as cereal, bread, pasta, grains, fruits, and vegetables. Carbohydrates provide the main source of energy for the body.

CHOLESTEROL: A fatty substance in the body found in the blood. Too much of it can clog arteries and cause heart damage.

COLLAGEN: The basic protein substance of bone, cartilage, tendon, and skin, as well as all other connective tissue. It can be converted to gelatin by boiling.

COMPRESSION FRACTURE: A collapsed fracture of a bone in the vertebra or spine.

CONJUGATED ESTROGEN: This is the generic name for Premarin™ and PremPro™. Conjugated estrogens are made in the laboratory. Natural estrogens are usually obtained from plant sources and are often available in health food stores.

CORTICAL BONE: The hard, dense outer layer of bone.

CORTICOSTEROID: A group of hormones produced in the adrenal gland. The name also applies to medicines that duplicate the activity of these hormones. These are anti-inflammatory medications and are used to treat arthritis and asthma, among other medical conditions. **Prednisone** (Deltasone™, Meticorten™, Orasone™, Prelone™) and **cortisone** (Cortone™) are examples of this type of drug.

COX-2 INHIBITOR: Abbreviation for cyclooxygenase inhibitor, a nonsteroidal anti-inflammatory drug (NSAID) used to relieve arthritis and other conditions. These include Celebrex™ and Vioxx™.

DEMENTIA: An acquired organic mental disorder characterized by loss of intellectual abilities severe enough to interfere with social or occupational functioning.

DUAL-ENERGY X-RAY ABSORPTIOMETRY (DEXA): This is the most accurate BMD test available. Photon beams are aimed at your hip, spine, or wrist. The denser (healthier) your bone, the less energy passes through it. It is painless, quick, and uses one tenth of the radiation used by standard X ray.

ELECTROLYTES: Chemicals in the body that help regulate the balance of fluids and other cell functions.

ENZYME: A protein or conjugated protein produced by a living organism, which acts as a catalyst for biochemical reactions.

ERT: The acronym for estrogen replacement therapy.

ESOPHAGUS: The tube connecting the mouth to the stomach. Sometimes called the swallowing tube.

ESTRACE™: The trade name for an FDA-approved oral medication to prevent osteoporosis. It is manufactured by Bristol-Myers Squibb.

ESTRADERM™: The trade name for the 17 beta-estradiol patch approved by the FDA to prevent osteoporosis. It is made by Novartis Pharmaceuticals.

ESTRATAB™: The trade name for an FDA-approved esterified estrogen to help prevent osteoporosis. It is made by Solvay Pharmaceuticals.

ESTROGENS: A class of sex hormones responsible for the development and maintenance of secondary female sex characteristics and control of the changes in the reproductive cycle. They are important in maintaining bone density.

EVISTA™: The trade name for raloxifene, a selective estrogen receptor modulator (SERM) approved by the FDA for the prevention and treatment of osteoporosis in women. It is made by Eli Lilly & Co.

EXERCISE: Rapid movement and exertion of the body to promote firmness and muscle development. Continuous exercise is very important for the prevention of osteoporosis.

FAMILY HISTORY: A history of osteoporosis in the immediate family, especially the mother and father. It is often signaled by a hip, wrist, or spine fracture when the relative was fifty or older. People with a family history of osteoporosis are more likely than others to develop it themselves.

FDA: The acronym for the U.S. Food and Drug Administration. They must test and approve all medications sold in the United States.

FIBER: The indigestible part of some fruits, vegetables, and whole grains that helps maintain healthy functioning of the bowels and prevents constipation.

FLUORIDE: A compound believed to stimulate the growth of new bone by increasing the activity of osteoblasts, the bone builders. As yet, fluoride has not been approved by the FDA for the treatment of osteoporosis.

FORTEO™: The trade name for the recently FDA-approved synthetic parathyroid hormone teriparatide, used for the treatment of osteoporosis in both men and women. It is the only medication that actually builds new bone and it must be given by injection. The manufacturer is Eli Lilly & Co.

FOSAMAX™: The trade name for alendronate, a bisphosphonate approved by the FDA to treat osteoporosis in postmenopausal women. It is manufactured by Merck & Co.

FRACTURE: A break in the bone. A bone fracture is often the first indication a person gets that she or he may have osteoporosis.

GEL: A combination of liquid and solid that creates a substance with a texture similar to glue or jelly. Gels are often used in medications in capsule form.

HIGH-DENSITY LIPOPROTEIN (HDL): A type of cholesterol that carries fatty deposits to the liver for elimination from the body. HDL is often referred to as "good cholesterol," because if these fatty deposits are not eliminated and instead build up in the body, they can cause heart disease or stroke.

HORMONE REPLACEMENT THERAPY (HRT): A general term that applies to all types of estrogen replacement therapy (ERT), the difference being that HRT is given along with progesterone. It was often prescribed to help postmenopausal women manage the symptoms of menopause. Women's Health Initiative study results published in July 2002 raised questions about its safety, and many women stopped using it. In October 2002, the NIH and the FDA suggested the term be changed to hormone therapy (HT) to reflect the nature of its use more accurately.

HOT FLASH: A symptom of menopause in which a woman suddenly feels hot, begins to perspire, and may experience a reddening of the face and neck. Hormone therapy has been used to treat hot flashes.

HYPERTENSION (HIGH BLOOD PRESSURE): A person's blood pressure is considered high when the systolic pressure is above 140 mm Hg, and the diastolic pressure is above 90 mm Hg, or both.

HYSTERECTOMY: An operation in which a woman's uterus is surgically removed. Women who have had hysterectomies can safely take unopposed estrogen without increasing their risk of breast cancer.

IMMUNE SYSTEM: The substances and cells in the body that protect us from infection and disease.

INSULIN: A hormone produced by the pancreas that helps regulate the level of blood sugar (glucose) in the body.

LOW-DENSITY LIPOPROTEIN (LDL): The type of cholesterol that builds up in the body and can cause heart disease or stroke. LDL is often referred to as "bad cholesterol."

LUPUS: A disorder of the immune system that causes inflammation of the connective tissue.

MACRONUTRIENT: A vitamin or mineral required in large amounts for the normal nutrition, growth, and development of an organism.

MAGNESIUM: An essential mineral in calcium absorption, nerve impulse transmission, muscle contraction, and the formation of bones and teeth. It should be taken in a 2:1 ratio with calcium; that is, one part magnesium for every two parts calcium.

MENOPAUSE: The completion of the period when a woman's ovaries stop functioning and her menstrual periods end. Menopause is considered complete when a woman has not had a menstrual period for a year.

MIACALCIN™: The trade name for salmon calcitonin in nasal spray form. It is approved by the FDA for treatment of osteoporosis in postmenopausal women and is manufactured by Sandoz Pharmaceuticals.

MICRONUTRIENT: A vitamin or mineral that is needed in minute amounts to ensure the healthy growth and metabolism of an organism.

MILLIGRAM (mg): a unit of weight in the metric system used to describe dosage of medication. 1,000 micrograms (mcg) equal 1 milligram and 1,000 milligrams equal 1 gram.

NORMAL BONE MASS: The description of bone density that is within one standard deviation of the mean bone mass for a normal, young adult. This would be measured as a T-score above −1 standard deviation.

OGEN™: The trade name for piperazine estrone sulfate, an FDA-approved medication for the treatment of osteoporosis. It is made by Upjohn.

OSSIFICATION: The process by which cartilage is converted into hard bone.

OSTEOARTHRITIS: Arthritis caused by long-term stress on the joints. It is common in people over sixty-five.

OSTEOBLAST: The bone builders, cells that form bone.

OSTEOPENIA: A condition in which bone mass is lower than normal, but not low enough to be called osteoporosis. A T-score between −1 and −2.5 indicates osteopenia.

OSTEOPOROSIS: A progressive bone disease characterized by low bone mass and continuing deterioration of bone. This often leads to fracture and loss of height. A T-score from a bone mineral density test that is at or below −2.5 standard deviations indicates osteoporosis.

PAGET'S DISEASE: A disorder in which the bone does not form properly, causing bones to become weak, thick, and deformed.

PEAK BONE MASS: The maximum bone mass that is achieved in the skeleton, usually by the age of eighteen in women and twenty in men.

PERIPHERAL FRACTURES: Bone breaks that occur not in the spine or vertebra, but in the hip, wrist, forearm, ankle, foot, rib, and sternum.

PHYTOCHEMICALS: Substances in food that provide the color-giving pigments. Some of them are particularly effective in decreasing cholesterol, and others are powerful antioxidants.

PREMARIN™: The trade name for conjugated estrogen, an oral estrogen therapy approved by the FDA for treatment and prevention of osteoporosis. It is produced by Wyeth Ayerst.

PROGESTIN/PROGESTERONE: The female sex hormone that is taken along with estrogen to help reduce the risk of endometrial cancer in women who have an intact uterus.

PROTEINS: Large molecules made up of amino acids that are essential in forming the basis of body structures such as hair and skin, and chemicals such as enzymes and hormones. Too much protein in the diet can cause a loss of calcium.

RALOXIFENE: The generic name for Evista™, a selective estrogen receptor modulator (SERM).

REMODELING: The process whereby new bone is formed by the bone-builders (osteoblasts), and old bone is cleared away (resorbed) by the bone clearers (osteoclasts).

RESISTANCE TRAINING: The exercise method for strengthening muscle by using weights or elastic bands to increase the force of the contraction of the muscle. By creating consistent force on the bone in this way, bone density increases.

RESORPTION: The breakdown of bone implemented by the osteoclasts.

RHEUMATOID ARTHRITIS: A type of arthritis caused by swelling and inflammation of the joints.

SD: Standard deviation from the norm. This is a measurement used in assessing the T-score in a bone density test.

SEROTONIN: A chemical that transmits nerve impulses that cause blood vessels to constrict. Serotonin levels in the brain also affect mood, so that selective serotonin reuptake inhibitors (SSRIs) are used to treat depression. These SSRIs include: Celexa™, Luxov™, Paxil™, Prozac™, and Zoloft™.

SINGLE-ENERGY X-RAY ABSORPTIOMETRY (SEXA): A diagnostic test used to measure bone density in peripheral sites, not the spine and hip.

STATINS: Medications used to lower cholesterol. Some help lower triglyceride levels and raise the good cholesterol HDL levels. Statins include: Baycol™, Lescol™, Lipitor™, Mevacor™, Pravachol™, and Zocor™.

STEROIDS: A group of synthesized chemical compounds that mimic the activity of hormones. They include cortisone and prednisone.

SUPPLEMENTS: Something added to what a person eats to make up for a lack in that person's diet. Vitamins and minerals often come in supplement form.

SYNTHETIC: Produced from a chemical process rather than a natural source, as in conjugated estrogens.

TESTOSTERONE: A sex hormone or androgen produced in men and women. In men it encourages the growth of bone and muscle. Testosterone replacement therapy (TRT) works for men with osteoporosis caused by low testosterone levels. It has no affect on bone mineral density in men with normal testosterone levels.

THYROID: A small gland in the front of the neck that produces natural hormones that control the energy functions of the body. The thyroid releases these chemicals into the body.

THYROID MEDICATIONS: Medications used to increase the amount of thyroid hormone in the body when the thyroid gland is not producing enough, causing a condition called hypothyroidism. These medications include: Armour™ Thyroid, Cytomel™, Eltroxin™, Levo-T™, Levothyroid™, Levoxine™, Levoxyl™, Synthroid™, Thyrolar™, and others. These medications can sometimes interfere with calcium absorption.

TOXIC: Poisonous. A substance that is capable of causing illness or even death, especially by chemical means.

TRANSDERMAL: Through the skin.

TRABECULAR BONE: The soft, spongy inner core of the bone.

T-SCORE: Used to describe bone mineral density (BMD). It refers to the number of standard deviations above or below the mean for normal, young adults.

ULTRASOUND DENSITOMETRY: A diagnostic test used to assess the bone density in the knee or ankle.

VITAMIN D: A fat-soluble vitamin essential to the absorption of calcium. We get it through the foods we eat, or we make it ourselves when our skin is exposed to the ultraviolet rays of the sun, and our bodies are able to store it. We need between 400 IU and 800 IU per day.

Z-SCORE: Used in bone mineral density (BMD) tests, it measures the number of standard deviations above or below the mean for women or men of your age.

ACKNOWLEDGMENTS

So many people have generously donated their time, energy, enthusiasm, and expertise to the creation of *Beautiful Bones Without Hormones*, it is difficult to come up with a way to thank them adequately. The following, in alphabetical order, is a list of some of our most valuable allies, people to whom we are eternally grateful:

Norma Bonaiuto, a gifted assistant who worked tirelessly and cheerfully to help us put this book together

Fredrica Friedman, our brilliant, perceptive, super-supportive literary agent who put us together in the first place

Abby Gerstein, an inspired nutritionist and founder of Nutritional Solutions, who spent hours, days, weeks checking all the nutritional information in this book and who contributed some of her own favorite high-calcium recipes

Elizabeth Lee Kelly, an exceptionally gifted young artist who created the beautiful drawings for the book

Dr. Joseph Lane, attending orthopedic surgeon and chief of the Metabolic Bone Service at the Hospital for Special Surgery, for his continuing good counsel, advice, and generous support

Erin Moore, our editor extraordinaire, for her stunning intelligence, efficiency, and cheerful disposition, not to mention her unfailing enthusiasm and support

The National Osteoporosis Foundation, especially Harriet Shapiro for their time, enthusiastic support, and generous contributions to the accuracy of this book

Rebecca and Peter Rosow, great pals and great sports who posed for the exercise photographs in the book

Dr. Linda Russell, attending internist and associate chief of the Metabolic Bone Service at the Hospital for Special Surgery, for her tireless support, advice, and encouragement

William Shinker, our fine publisher who had the wisdom and insight to see the urgent need for this book, and the graciousness to be supportive every step of the way

Ian Spanier, the gifted photographer who styled and photographed the models for the exercise section of the book

And to our families and dear friends who suffered through hours of osteoporosis talk and recipe testing and tasting. We love you all!

—LEON ROOT, M.D.   —BETTY KELLY SARGENT

INDEX

Abdominal Crunches exercise, 236–37
Active Knee Extension exercise, 240
acupuncture, 256
Adductor Stretch, 232a
aerobic exercises, 243–57
  balance, 247–248
  cycling, 249–51
  dancing, 251
  swimming, 248–49
  tai chi, 252–53
  tai chi chi, 253–54
  walking, 245–47
  water aerobics, 249
  Yoga, 251–52
African Americans, 22, 32, 33–34, 56–57
age, 28–30, 31
  BMD test and, 36
  calcium requirements by, 79
  exercise and, 29
  -related osteoporosis, 17–18
  young people and osteoporosis, 52–53
AI (Adequate Intake), 129
alcohol, 27, 38–39, 102, 152–53
Alcoholics Anonymous, 152–53
alendronate (Fosamax), 58–61
Alzheimer's disease, 13, 64
amenorrhea, 52–52
American Dietetic Association, 158
anemia, 56, 101
  sickle-cell, 33
anorexia nervosa, 19, 27, 53
antacids
  with aluminum, 19, 42–43
  non-aluminum, 43
antibiotics, 44, 90
anticoagulants, 44
anticonvulsants, 43
antioxidants, 115
aoledronic acid (Zometa), 62
Asians, 32, 33
aspirin, 61, 62
astronauts, 17
avocado, 135

balance exercises, 247–48
Barnes, Ronnie, 255
Barrett-Connor, Dr. Elizabeth, 13
Begley, Sharon, 26
Bent Knee Standing exercise, 248
berries, 223
beta-carotene, 103
Biceps and Triceps exercises, 235
biotin, 113
bisphosphonates, 59–62, 67
blackstrap molasses, 223
bleeding, 101
blood clots, 12, 13, 63, 75
blood pressure, 75, 78
blood-thinners, 44
BMP2 gene, 26
body type, 31–32
bomb calorimeter, 160
bone marrow diseases, 19
bone mineral density (BMD) tests, 5
  CAT scan, 46
  DEXA, 45
  importance of, 24
  insurance coverage, 6
  meaning of low, 7–10
  risk factors and, 27
  SEXA, 45–46
  QUS, 46
  types of, 5–6, 44–46
  when to get, 36–37, 47
bones. *See also* medications, bone-building;
    osteoporosis; *and* calcium *and other specific nutrients*
  achieving optimal mass, in growth years,
    16–17
  aerobic exercises for, 243–57
  age of maximum density, 16
  "bank," of calcium, 80
  -building medications, 58–70
  calcium and, 73–98
  children and, 308–11
  cortical, 15
  defined, 7

bones (*cont.*)
  eating program to maximize strength of,
    218–24
  ethnicity and, 32–35
  foods that help, 131–44
  foods to avoid, 148–55
  foods to cut down on, 144–48
  formation of, 7
  fractures, 13, 34
  HRT/ERT and, 11–12
  job of, 7
  loss, 7, 11, 30–31
  low mass, 32–35, 74
  medications to build, 58–70
  menu plans for, 157–217
  minerals essential for, 114, 119–26
  normal mass, 10
  reason for break down of, 16–17
  recipes for, 259–318
  remodeling cycle of, 8–9
  resorption, alcohol and, 39
  tissue types, 15
  trabecular, 15
  vitamin D and, 99–109
  vitamins for, 110–18
  weight-bearing exercise for, 227–42
bone tumors (osteosarcomas), 67
boron, 81, 92, 114
  benefits and sources of, 119–21
bread, calcium-fortified, 223, 224
breast cancer, 11, 12, 13, 14, 16, 75, 77
breathing exercises, 230
Brody, Jane E., 73
bulimia malabsorption, 19
B vitamins, 116–18. *See also specific vitamins*

caffeine, 27, 39–41, 148–50
  amounts of, in beverages, 40–41, 150
caffeinism, 148
calcitonin, 58, 59
  how to take, and side effects, 65–66
  nasal spray (Miacalcin), 66
calcitriol, 103–4
calcium, 20, 73–98, 113, 114. *See also* cal-
    cium supplements *and specific types*
  absorption of, 28–30, 80, 87, 94–97
    boosting, 110–30
  adding, to diet tips, 222–24
  African Americans and, 33–34
  alcohol and, 38, 152–153
  balance, 38
  benefits of, 75–78
  bones and, 81–82
  boron and, 120
  caffeine and, 39, 40, 148–50
  children and, 308–9

  in dairy products, 83–84, 132–34
  defined, 74–76
  diet facts, 132, 134, 141
  elemental, 94–97
  experts on, 73–76
  facts, 76, 78, 79, 80, 86, 87, 95
  in fish and shellfish, 142–43
  food sources of, 82–87, 131–48
  in fruits, 135–37
  gender and, 31
  in grains, 143–44
  Hispanics and, 35
  how much to take, 6, 78–81
  importance of, 24, 78
  in legumes, 141–42
  low, as risk factor, 41
  in meat and poultry, 145–46
  in nondairy foods, 85–86
  in nuts and seeds, 140
  recipes high in, 261–319
  risk factors and, 27
  salt and, 153–54
  in vegetables, 138–40
  vitamin D and, 105
  vitamins and minerals required with, 81
  youth needs, 16
calcium carbonate, 93–95, 95, 97
calcium citrate, 93–94, 95, 97
calcium deficiency, 74
  dangers of, 77–78
  14-day High-Calcium Diet for, 74
  7-day High-Calcium Diet for Lactose-
    Intolerant for, 74
  7-day High-Calcium Diet for Vegetarians
    for, 74
  symptoms, 79, 80
calcium gluconate, 97
calcium lactate, 97
calcium supplements
  combining with other vitamins and min-
    erals, 54–55
  elemental, 96
  how much to take at one time, 93
  recommended daily amounts, 98
  supplements to take with, 93–94
  type to take, 93–97
Calf-Muscle Stretch, 230–31
calories, 159–60
calorimetry, 160
cancer. *See also* specific types
  calcium and, 75
  vegetables that fight, 138
carbohydrates
  complex, 110
  energy in, 158–59
  simple or refined, 110

carotenoids, 103
CAT or CT scan (Computerized Axial Tomography), 46
Caucasians (whites), 32, 33, 34
cell membrane, 75
cervical cancer, 16
cheese, 221–23
children, 16–18, 76
  high-calcium recipes for, 308–19
chiropractic treatment, 256
chloride, 113, 114
cholecalciferol, 104
cholesterol, 147
Cioppa, Jeme Mosca, 244
coffee, 40, 149, 222
collagen, 75, 81–82, 125
colon cancer, 12, 13, 74–77
color, in foods, 219–20
compact bone (cortical bone), 81
copper, 81, 92, 114
  benefits and sources of, 121–22
cortical content, of bones, 15, 21
corticosteroids, 19, 27, 38–39, 42
Coumadin, 44
cruciferous vegetables, 138
Cushing syndrome, 19
cycling, 249–51
cystic fibrosis, 19

dancing, 251
dark-green leafy vegetables, 82, 139–wwwwwwwwwwww40
Davy, Sir Humphry, 74
death, leading causes of, 50
DeCode Genetics, 26
Deep Breathing exercise, 230
Delmas, Dr. Pierre, 25
depression, 19
DEXA (dual-energy X-ray absorptiometry), 45
diabetes mellitus, 19
diarrhea, 27
diary products, 82–84, 131–34
  calcium in, 132–34, 147–48
  copper in, 122
dibasic calcium phosphate, 97
diet
  14-day High-Calcium, 74, 157–89
  guidelines, government website on, 129
  long-term eating program to maximize bone strength, 218–24
  7-day High-Calcium, for Lactose-Intolerant, 74, 84, 86, 190–203
  7-day High-Calcium, for Vegetarians, 74, 84, 204–17
  ten tips for healthy bones, 156

thirty tips to add calcium to every day, 222–24
tips, 82, 83, 84, 86, 87
tips for kids, 309
dilantin, 19
diuretics, 43
  loop, 19, 43, 69
  non-loop, 69
  thiazide, 122
DRI (Dietary Reference Intake), 129, 130
DRV (Daily Reference Value), 130
DV (Daily Value), 130

EAR (Estimate Average Requirement), 129–30
eggs, 134
electrolytes, 114
elliptical trainers, 254
endocrine conditions, 19
energy, 158, 160
enzymes, 126
epiphysis of bone, 81
ergocalciferol, 104
estradiol, 38
estren, 69
estrogen
  boron and, 120
  estren, 69
  natural, 69
  for osteoporosis, 59, 64–65
  preventing bone loss and, xiv–xv
  SERMS to mimic, 55
  smoking and, 151–152
estrogen-progesterone products, 65
estrogen replacement therapy (ERT or ET), xiv, 13, 14
ethnicity, 32–35
etidronate (Didronel), 62
European Union, 33
exercise, 6
  aerobic, 227, 243–54
  age and, 29
  amenorrhea from too much, 19, 52–53
  benefit of, 243–44
  fifteen-minute morning routine, 229–42
  floor, 236–39
  gender and, 31
  importance of, 24, 254
  lack of, as risk factor, 37
  personal training vs. physical therapy, 255–56
  sitting, 240–42
  strengthening, 232–36
  stretching and breathing, 229–32
  ten-point system, 228–29
  weight-bearing, 227–42

fall-proofing
  home, 51–52
  yourself, 52
family history, 35
fats, 146–48
  defined, 111
  energy in, 158, 160
  high-calcium diet to decrease, 158
  metabolism, calcium to aid, 75, 76
  polyunsaturated, saturated, and mono-
    unsaturated, 147
figs, dried, 135
fish and shellfish, 82, 142–43
fish oils, 104
floor exercises, 236–39
fluids, defined, 110
fluoride, 68
folic acid (vitamin B9), 92, 102, 112
  benefits and sources of, 117–18
Food and Drug Administration (FDA), xiv,
    40, 58
  website, 129
foods, 131–56. *See also* diet; Recipe Index
  boron sources, 121
  calcium content
    dairy chart, 83–84
    nondairy chart, 85–86
  calcium sources
    best, 131–44
    not so good, 144–48
    terrible, 148–55
  copper sources, 122
  dairy, 129–34
  fats and oils, 146–48
  fish and shellfish, 142–43
  fruits, 135–37
  grains, 143–44
  grocery list, 221
  high in calcium, 80, 82–87
  label terms, 129–30
  legumes, 141
  magnesium sources, 123
    chart, 88
  to maximize bone strength, 218–24
  meats, 145–46
  nuts and seeds, 140
  oxalates in, 87
  phosphorus sources, 125
  phytochemicals and color in, 219–20
  processed, 125, 153–54
  quick, high-calcium, for kids, 309–11
  silica sources, 126
  six elements of, 110–12
  ten diet tips for, 156
  30 tips to add calcium to everyday,
    222–24

to-do list, 221
vegetables, 138–40
vitamin B6 sources, 116
vitamin B9 (folic acid) sources, 118
vitamin B12 sources, 117
vitamin C sources, 115
vitamin D sources, 115
  chart, 89, 106–8
  fortified chart, 108
vitamin K sources, 119
  chart, 91
zinc sources, 127
  chart, 92
Forteo. *See* parathyroid hormone
Fosamax. *See* alendronate
14-day High-Calcium Diet, 74, 157–89
  menus, 162–89
free radicals, 115
fruits, 135–37, 223
  calcium list, 135–37
  color in, 219–20
  facts, 137

Gaucher's disease, 19
gender, 30–31
genetic factors, 26
gonadotropin-releasing hormone agonists,
    19
grains, 143–44
gums, 21

Haber, Karen, 249
Hamstring Stretch, 231
Heaney, Dr. Robert, 40, 149
heart, 75
  attack, 11, 13, 16, 102
  disease, 12, 13
Heparin, 44
hereditary diseases, 19
hip, 19, 20, 21
hip fracture, 13, 30, 31
  worldwide incidence of, 23–24, 35, 57
Hippocrates, 218
Hispanics, 32, 33, 34–34
homocystein, 102
hormone replacement therapy (HRT or
    HT), xiv
  alcohol and, 38
  alendronate as substitute for, 60–61
  dangers of, 14
  how to stop, 65
  myth about not being on, 55
  preventing osteoporosis without, xiv
  pros and cons of, 11–14
  smoking and, 151–52
  vitamin D and, 103–4

Hospital for Special Surgery (HSS), 67, 244, 250, 251, 255
hot flashes, 63, 120
hydrochlorothiazide, 69
hypercalciuria, 19
hyperparathyroidism, 19
hyperthyroidism, 42
hypogonadism, 19
hypophosphatasia, 19
hypothyroidism, 42
hysterectomies, 14

indoles, 138
insomnia, 75
International Osteoporosis Foundation (IOF), 25
ipriflavone, 69

Journal of the American College of Nutrition, 76
Journal of the American Medical Association (JAMA), 13
Journal of the National Cancer Institute, 77
juice, orange or grapefruit, 86, 221–24

kidney, 105
Klinefeltner's syndrome, 19
Knee Bend exercise, Modified, 233

lactase enzymes, 132
lactose intolerance, 33–34, 57
  dairy products for, 132, 134
  7-day High-Calcium Diet for 74, 84, 86, 190–203
leg cramps, 63
legumes, 141
Li, Dr. Christopher, 14
lithium, 19, 44
liver, 105
Lupkin, Dr. Martin, 73
lupus, 19, 33, 56

macrominerals, 113
macular degeneration, 13, 115
magnesium, 20, 113, 114
  alcohol and, 38
  benefits and sources of, 87–88, 122–23
  boron and, 120
  recommended daily supplement, 98
  taking, with calcium, 81
mammograms, 14
manganese, 92, 114
  benefits and sources of, 123–24
Marching in Place exercise, 235–36
massage, 256
meat, 145–46

medications, bone-building, 50–51, 58–70
  bishpsphonates category, 59–62
  calcitonin, 65–66
  estren, 69
  estrogens, 64–65
  fluoride, 68
  natural estrogens, 69
  non-loop diuretics, 69
  parathyroid hormone (PTH), 66–67
  SERMS, 55, 63–64
  statins, 68
medications, causing osteoporosis, 18–19, 41–44
Melton, L.J., 35
men
  calcium and, 77
  ethnicity and, 33
  leading risk factors list, 54
  myth of not having osteoporosis, 53–54
  NOF figures on osteoporosis in, 31
  osteoporosis risk and, 7
  recommended diet and vitamins for, 54
  testosterone levels and, 29
menopause, 11, 13, 120
  bone loss rate and, 7
  early surgical, 19
  risk factors and, 26
  weight loss and, 32, 76
metabolic diseases, 19
methlysanthines, 148
methotrexate, 19, 44
Mexican Americans, 34
micrograms (mcg), 114
milk, 82–84. *See also* dairy products
  adding, to diet, 222
  nonfat dry milk, 222, 223
  skim vs. whole, 132
  vitamin D fortified, 104
milligrams (mg), 114
minerals. *See also* calcium; vitamin and mineral supplements; *and other specific minerals*
  benefits and sources of, 119–27
  chelated, 88
  defined, 111
  Dr. Root's recommendations chart, 128
  essential for bone health list, 111, 114
  essential for human health list, 113–14
  how much to take, 128–29
multivitamin, 92–93

National Cancer Institute, 13
National Center for Health Statistics, 49
National Health and Nutrition Examination Survey, 34

National Institutes of Health (NIH), 6, 56, 79, 130
National Osteoporosis Foundation (NOF), 3, 30
National Soft Drink Association, 40
Neck-to-Foot Bridge exercise, 237
Neilsen, Dr. Forest, 120
nerves, 75, 101
New England Journal of Medicine, 102, 105
nonsteroidal anti-inflammatory drugs (NSAIDs), 60
NordicTrack, 254
Nurses' Health Study, 13, 102, 118–19, 151
Nutrient Database for Standard Reference, 132
Nutrition and Your Health, 129
nuts and seeds, 140

oatmeal, 222
Office of Dietary Supplements (ODS), 130
oils, 146–48
ORAC (oxygen radical absorbance capacity), 219–20
osteoarthritis, 244
osteoblasts, 8–9, 16, 82
  age and, 30
  alcohol and, 39, 152
  magnesium and, 88
osteocalcin, 118
osteoclasts, 8–9, 16, 30, 82
osteocytes, 8–9
osteogenesis imperfecta, 19
osteomalacia 38, 62
osteopenia, 10
osteoporosis. *See also* bones; calcium; medications, bone-building
  BMD test for, 5–10, 24, 36–38, 44–47
  danger and prevalence of, xiv–xv, 3–5
  death from, 10, 49–50
  defined, 3–25, 82
  diagnosis of, 5, 10, 26, 81 (*see also* bone mass density test)
  as epidemic, 3–4, 24
  exercise and, 244
  facts, 3, 5, 6, 7, 10, 16, 17
  fractures, annual number, 16
  idiopathic, 18, 29
  medications for, 58–70
  primary, 17–18
  quiz for risk, 26–27
  risk factors
    changeable, 35–47
    unchangeable, 28–35
  secondary, 17, 18–19
  10 myths about, 48–57

  three steps to prevent, 24
  type I, 17–18, 29
  type II, 18, 29
  U.S. statistics on, 21–22
  who is at risk for, and why, 25–47
  why we get, 20–21
  worldwide statistics on, 23–24, 34
Osteoporosis and Related Bone Disease National Resource Center, 56
osteoporosis myths
  "African-American women don't have," 56–57
  "calcium-rich foods and supplements, I'll be fine," 54–55
  "men don't have to worry about," 53–54
  "mother didn't have," 55–56
  "never killed anybody," 49–50
  "normal part of aging," 50
  "not much I can do about it," 50–52
  "not on HRT, I'll probably get," 55
  "old lady's disease," 48–49
  "too young to worry about," 52–53
ovarian cancer, 13, 16
ovary removal, 19
oxalates, 86–87, 138

pamidronate, 62
parathyroid hormone (PTH), 38, 39, 59, 88, 123
  how to take, and side effects, 66–67
perimenopause, 11
personal training, 255–56
phenobarbitol, 19
phosphorus, 20, 92, 113, 114
  benefits and sources of, 124–25
physical therapy, 255–56
physis of bone, 81
phytates, 141
phytochemicals, 219–20
PMS, calcium and, 77
postmenopausal osteoporosis (Type I), 17
potassium, 113, 114
pregnancy, 19, 78, 81, 102
premenopausal women, 77
Prempro, 12, 13
Prevention's Giant Book of Health Facts, 38
prolactinoma, 19
Prone Leg Lift exercise, 238–39
Prone Upper-Body Life exercise, 239
protein, 110, 158
  too much, 154–55

QUS (quantitative ultrasound), 46

raloxifene hydrochloride (Evista), 58, 59, 63–64

RDA (Recommended Dietary Allowance), 129, 130
remodeling, of bone, 82
renal insufficiency, 19
resorption, 16, 7
retinoids, 103
rheumatoid arthritis, 19
rickets, 19
Riggs, B.L., 35
risedronate sodium, 59, 61–62
risk factors, 25–47
  age, 28–30
  alcohol, 38–39
  BMD test and, 36–38
  body type, 31–32
  caffeine, 39–41
  changeable, 35–47
  ethnicity, 32–35
  family history, 35
  gender, 30–31
  how to start reducing, 47
  lack of exercise, 37
  low body weight, 41
  low calcium and vitamin D, 41
  medications as, 41–44
  men and, 54
  quiz to assess, 26–27
  smoking, 37
  unchangeable, 28–35

salmon, 223, 224
salt, 153–54
Sandler, Dr. Robert, 76
sardines, 223
selenium, 92
sequential progestin, 14
SERMs (selective estrogen receptor modulators), 55, 59, 63–64
7-day High-Calcium Diet for Lactose-Intolerant, 74, 84, 86
  menus, 190–203
7-day High-Calcium Diet for Vegetarians, 74, 84
  menus, 204–17
SEXA (single-energy S-ray absorptiometry), 45–46
Shoulder Strengthening exercise, 234
Side Leg Lifts exercise, 238
Side Stepping exercise, 248
silica, 114
  benefits and sources of, 125–26
silicon, 81, 92
Single Leg Standing exercise, 248
Sitting exercises, 240–42
smoking, 37, 151–52
sodium, 20, 113, 114

soft drinks, caffeine in, 40–41
soy, in diet, 69
spine, 19
StairMaster, 254
statins, 68
Steffansson, Kari, 26
steroids, 42
Stretching exercise, 229–30
stroke, 11, 12, 13, 16
strontium, 92
sugar, 154
sulfur, 113
sunlight, 100–101
swimming, 248–49

Tai chi, 247, 251, 252–53
Tai chi chi, 253–53
tamoxifen, 64
Tandem Walking, 247
tea, 40
teriparatide (Forteo), 67. *See also* parathyroid hormone (PTH)
testosterone, 27, 29, 38, 120
tetracycline, 44
Thigh-Clencher exercise, 241
Thigh Lift exercise, 241
Thigh-Spreader exercise, 242
thyroid medication, 19, 27, 42
Thys-Jacobs, Dr. Susan, 77
to-do list, 3-step everyday, 221
Toe Raises exercise, 232
tofu, 82, 142, 161
Tosi, Dr. Laura, 103
trabecular bone, 15, 21, 81
trace minerals, 113
trans fats, 147
tribasic calcium phosphate, 97
t-score, 10, 46
tuna, 223
Turner's syndrome, 19

UC Berkeley Wellness Letter Book, 143, 154
UL (Tolerable Upper Intake Level), 129
United States, 21–23
Up and Down exercise, 247–48
Upper-Back Strengthening exercise, 234
uterine cancer, 14, 16

vegetables
  calcium list, 138–40
  color in, and phytochemicals, 219–20
vegetarians, 155
  7-day High-Calcium Diet for 74, 84, 204–17
VersaClimber, 254

vitamin A (retinol), 102, 112
  toxic levels of, 102–3
  type to take, 103
vitamin B1 (thiamine), 102, 112
vitamin B2 (riboflavin), 112
vitamin B3 (niacin), 102, 112
vitamin B5 (pantothenic acid), 112
vitamin B6 (pyridoxine), 92, 102, 112
  benefits and sources of, 116
vitamin B9. *See* folic acid
vitamin B12 (cobalamin), 92, 102, 113
  benefits and sources of, 117
vitamin C, 92, 112
  benefits and sources of, 115
  taking, with calcium, 81
vitamin D, 99–109, 112
  absorption of, 104
  age and, 29
  alcohol and, 38
  anticonvulsants, 43
  benefits and sources of, 89–90, 99–104
  caffeine and, 40
  calcium absorption and, 102
  D2, 90, 104
  D3, 90, 104, 105
  daily recommended intake, 98,
    114–15
  deficiency, 102
  food labels and, 106
  food sources of, 106–8
  fruits and, 137
  hormones and, 103–4
  how much to take, 104–8
  kidney and liver and, 105
  magnesium and, 88
  sunlight and, 100
  supplements, 104, 106, 108–9
  taking, with calcium, 54–55, 81, 93–94
  vitamin A and, 102–103
  youth and, 16
vitamin E, 102, 112
vitamin K, 102, 112
  benefits and sources of, 90–91, 118–19
  food sources chart, 91
  recommended daily supplement, 98
  taking, with calcium, 81

vitamins, 114
  deficiency, 101
  essential, Dr. Root's recommendations
    chart, 128
  fat soluble, 112
  how much to take, 128–29
  required for bone health list, 111
  thirteen essential to human health list,
    112–13
  water soluble, 112–13
vitamins and mineral supplements. *See also*
    minerals; *and specific vitamins and
    minerals*
  daily recommendations for bones, 98
  daily requirements chart, 92–93
  label terms, 130–31

walking, 244–47
Walking Backward exercise, 248
Walton, Bill, 121–22
Warren, Dr. Russell, 255
water, 161
water aerobics, 249
weight
  loss, 32, 76
  osteoporosis and, 32, 41
weight-loss medications, 102
women
  ethnicity and, 32–35
  osteoporosis and, 30–31
Women's Health Initiative (WHI), xiv, 11–
    14
World Health Organization (WHO), 10,
    46, 57
"Worldwide Problem of Osteoporosis,
    The" (Riggs and Melton), 35
worldwide statistics, 23–24, 34, 35
wrist, 19, 20, 21

Yoga, 251–52
yogurt, 221–24

zinc, 81, 114
  benefits and sources of, 91–92, 126–27
  recommended daily supplement, 98
z-score, 10

RECIPE INDEX

Almonds
  Roasted Figs with Goat Cheese and, 284
  Spinach Salad with Blue Cheese and, 278
  Trout Amandine, 303–4
Apricot Ambrosia, 312
Arame
  Emerald Sea Salad, 275–76
  Salad, 274
Asparagus au Gratin, 285

Banana-Strawberry Surprise, 314
Beans
  Black Soup, 270–71
  Black-eyed Pea Salad, 275–76
Beet(s)
  and Orange Soup, 269–70
  and Beet Greens, Roasted with Rosemary Vinaigrette, 292–93
Berries and Melon with Lemon-Orange Sauce, 283–84
Black-eyed Pea Salad, 275–76
Blue Cheese
  Buttermilk Dressing, 281
  Vinaigrette, 280
  Warm Spinach Salad with Almonds and, 278
Broccoli
  and Cheese Casserole, 286–87
  with Creamy Garlic Sauce, 287–88
  and Penne Pasta, 298–99
  Soup, 271–72
Buttermilk
  Dill, Cucumber Dressing, 279–80
  Blue Cheese Dressing, 281
Butternut Squash Soup with Tofu and Chard, 272–73
Butterscotch Pudding, 318–19

Cabbage with Cauliflower au Gratin, 288–89
Chard, Butternut Squash Soup with Tofu and, 272–73

Cheese. *See also* Blue Cheese
  Bluefish with Yogurt and, 302
  Casserole, Broccoli and, 286–87
  Crackers, Crunchy, 316–17
  Dogs, 310
  Feta, Figs and Greens with, 290
  French Toast, 266–67
  Goat Cheese and Almonds, Roasted Figs with, 284
  Grits with Yogurt, 265–66
  Macaroni and, 315–16
  Pimento Spread, 318
  Quiche, Eggless Spinach and Mushroom, 267
  Sandwich
    Croque Monsieur 314–15
    Grilled Tomato and, 310
  Sauce, Mornay, 305
  Soufflé, 264–65
  Soup, Broccoli and, 271–72
  Straws, 317
  Tart, Sweet Onion, 268
  Tofu Breakfast Scramble, 269–70
Cherry-Mango Salsa, Wilted Mixed Greens, with 297–98
Crackers
  Cheese Straws, 317
  Crunchy Cheese, 316–17
Cream and Mint, Fresh Figs with, 281–82
Creamy Garlic Sauce, Broccoli with, 287–88
Croque Monsieur Sandwich, 314–15
Cucumber Buttermilk, Dill, Dressing, 279–80
Curried Greens, 289
Curry, Spinach and Tofu, 295

Dill, Cucumber, Buttermilk, Dressing, 279–80

Eggless Spinach and Mushroom Quiche, 267

Eggs, Scrumptious Scrambled, 310
Emerald Sea Salad, 275–76

Figs
  with Cream and Mint, 281–82
  with Goat Cheese and Almonds, Roasted, 284
  and Greens with Feta Cheese, 290
Fish
  Bluefish, Baked with Cheese and Yogurt, 302
  Salmon Cakes, Southern, 304
  Sardine Sauce, Pasta with, 300
  Trout Amandine, 303–4
  Tuna Melt, 309
  Sauces for, 305–7
French Toast, Cheesy, 266–67
Fruit, 281–84
  Fresh Frosty, 312–13
  Yogurt Parfait, 282

Garlic Sauce, Creamy, Broccoli with, 287–88
Gnocchi, Potato, 301–2
Greens
  Beet, with Roasted Beets and Rosemary Vinaigrette , 292–93
  Curried, 289
  Figs with Feta Cheese and, 290
  Mustard, with Raspberry Vinaigrette, 292
  Turnip, Tasty 297–98
  Wilted Mixed, with Mango-Cherry Salsa, 297–98
Grits, Cheese, with Yogurt, 265–66

Hijiki and Tofu Salad, 276
Hot Chocolate, 222
  Fluffy, 310

Kale
  au Gratin, 291
  and Potatoes with Portobello Mushrooms, Braised, 286

Lemon-Orange Sauce, Melon and Berries with, 283–84
Lentil, Red, Soup with Tofu and Wakame, 273

Macaroni and Cheese, 315–16
Mango-Cherry Salsa, Wilted Mixed Greens, with 297–98
Melon and Berries with Lemon-Orange Sauce, 283–84
Mint, Fresh Figs with Cream and, 281–82

Mornay Sauce, 305
Mushroom
  Quiche, Eggless Spinach and, 267
  Portobello, Braised Kale and Potatoes with, 286

Onion Tart, Sweet, 268
Orange
  -Lemon Sauce, Melon and Berries with, 283–84
  Sesame Sauce, 306
  Soup, Beet and, 269–70

Parfait
  Frozen Yogurt, 310
  Fruit Yogurt, 282
Pasta
  Fettuccini Alfredo, 299–300
  Macaroni and Cheese, 315–16
  Penne, Broccoli and, 298–99
  Potato Gnocchi, 301
  with Sardine Sauce, 300
Peanut Butter
  Delight, 313
  and Jelly Sandwich, 311
Pesto Sauce, 306
Pimento Cheese Spread, 318
Pizza, Mini, 310
Polenta, Spicy Swiss Chard with, 294–95
Potatoes
  Braised Kale with Portobello Mushrooms and, 286
  Gnocchi, 301
  Southern Scalloped, 293–94
Pudding, Butterscotch, 318–19

Quiche, Eggless Spinach and Mushroom, 267
Quinoa, Arame Salad, 274

Salad
  Arame, 274
  Black-eyed Pea, 275–76
  Emerald Sea, 275–76
  Southwestern-Style Tofu, 277
  Spinach with Blue Cheese and Almonds, Warm, 278
  Tofu and Hijiki, 276
  Watercress-Walnut, 278–79
Salad Dressing
  Buttermilk
    Dill, Cucumber 279–80
    Blue Cheese, 281
  Vinaigrette, 279
    Blue Cheese, 280
    Raspberry, 292
    Rosemary, 292–93

Salsa, Mango-Cherry, Wilted Mixed
    Greens, with 297–98
Sandwich
  Croque Monsieur, 314–15
  Grilled Cheese and Tomato, 310
  Peanut Butter and Jelly, 311
Sauce
  Creamy Garlic, 287–88
  Lemon-Orange, 283–84
  Mornay, 305
  Orange Sesame, 306
  Pesto, 306
  Sardine Pasta with, 300
Smoothie
  Apricot Ambrosia, 312
  Fresh Fruit Frosty, 312–13
  Peanut Butter Delight, 313
  Strawberry-Banana Surprise, 314
Soufflé, Cheese, 264–65
Soup
  Beet and Orange, 269–70
  Black Bean 270–71
  Broccoli, 271–72
  Butternut Squash with Tofu and Chard,
    272–73
  Red Lentil, with Tofu and Wakame, 273
Spinach
  Curry, Tofu and, 295
  Quiche, Eggless Mushroom and, 267
  Salad with Blue Cheese and Almonds,
    Warm, 278
Strawberry-Banana Surprise, 314

Swiss Chard
  with Polenta, Spicy, 294–95
  Supreme, 296

Tacos, Tasty, 310
Tart, Sweet Onion, 268
Tofu
  Breakfast Scramble, 269–70
  Curry, Spinach and, 295
  Quiche, Eggless Spinach and Mushroom,
    267
  Salad, Hijiki and, 276
  Soup
    Butternut Squash with Chard and,
      272–73
    Red Lentil with Wakame and,
      273
  Southwestern-Style, 277

Veggie Melt, 310

Wakame
  Emerald Sea Salad, 275–76
  Red Lentil Soup with Tofu and, 273
Watercress-Walnut Salad, 278–79

Yogurt
  Bluefish, Baked with Cheese and,
    302
  Cheese Grits with, 265–66
  Frozen Parfait, 310
  Fruit Parfait, 282

Dr. Leon Root, the author of the bestseller *Oh, My Aching Back*, is an orthopedic surgeon at the world-renowned Hospital for Special Surgery in New York, where he also serves as the director of Rehabilitation Medicine and director of the Back School Program. A professor of Clinical Orthopedics at the Weill College of Medicine, Cornell University, he is actively involved in teaching medical students and residents. He lives in New York City.

Betty Kelly Sargent is a veteran book and magazine editor who has worked for *The New Yorker* and as a senior editor at Dell Books, an executive editor at Delacorte Press, the editor in chief at William Morrow, and an editor at large for HarperCollins. She has originated and edited dozens of health and fitness books and has been published in many magazines, including *Cosmopolitan* (where she served as the book and fiction editor for fifteen years) and *Ladies Home Journal*. She lives in New York City.